DATE DUE

AP 19 00			
DE 6 01			

DEMCO 38-296

Severely Disturbed Youngsters and the Parental Alliance

Severely Disturbed Youngsters and the Parental Alliance

Jacquelyn Seevak Sanders, PhD
Barry L. Childress, MD
Editors

The Haworth Press, Inc.
New York • London • Norwood (Australia)

Severely Disturbed Youngsters and the Parental Alliance has also been published as *Residential Treatment for Children & Youth*, Volume 9, Number 4 1992.

The Haworth Press, Inc., 10 Alice Street, Binghamton, NY 13904-1580 USA

Library of Congress Cataloging-in-Publication Data

Severely disturbed youngsters and the parental alliance / Jacquelyn Seevak Sanders, Barry L. Childress, editors.
   p. cm.
   "Has also been published as Residential treatment for children & youth, volume 9, number 4, 1992."–T.p. verso.
   Includes bibliographical references.
   ISBN 1-56024-319-8 (alk. paper)
   1. Child psychotherapy–Congresses.2. Adolescent psychotherapy–Congresses.3. Mentally ill children–Family relationships–Congresses. 4. Countertransference (Psychology)–Congresses. I. Sanders, Jacquelyn Seevak. II. Childress, Barry L.
   [DNLM: 1. Countertransference (Psychology) 2. Mental Disorders–in adolescence. 3. Mental Disorders–in infancy & childhood. 4. Parent-Child Relations. W1 RE245V v. 9 no. 4 / WS 350 S498]
RJ504.S48   1992
618.92'8914–dc20
DNLM/DLC
for Library of Congress   92-1554
                                                                  CIP

Severely Disturbed Youngsters and the Parental Alliance

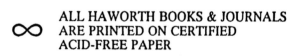

Severely Disturbed Youngsters and the Parental Alliance

CONTENTS

Severely Disturbed Youngsters and the Parental Alliance

ABOUT THE EDITORS

Jacquelyn Seevak Sanders, PhD, a licensed psychologist, has been Director of the Sonia Shankman Orthogenic School of the University of Chicago since 1973. She is also Senior Lecturer, Department of Education and Clinical Associate Professor, Department of Psychiatry, the University of Chicago. Dr. Sanders has authored a number of publications applying psychoanalytic theory to work with children in social settings, including *A Greenhouse for the Mind*, which deals primarily with education.

Barry L. Childress, MD, is a child analyst in private practice in Chicago, Illinois. He is on the faculty of the Chicago Institute for Psychoanalysis where he is Co-Director of the Child and Adolescent Psychotherapy Training Program (CAPT) and a member of the Child and Adolescent Psychoanalysis Committee. Dr. Childress has, for many years, consulted in the community, particularly with agencies serving families who have been involved with abused or neglected children.

Severely Disturbed Youngsters and the Parental Alliance

ABOUT THE CONTRIBUTORS

Efrain Bleiberg, MD, is Vice-President, Education, Research and Applications of the Menninger Foundation. He is also Director and Skillman Professor in Child Psychiatry at the Karl Menninger School of Psychiatry, and is an Instructor at the Topeka Institute for Psychoanalysis. He has written, presented, and published extensively, particularly on the development and treatment of narcissistic and other severe personality disorders in children. He may be written at the Menninger Clinic, Box 829, Topeka, KS 66601.

Daniel Frank, PhD, is Head of the Francis W. Parker Upper School, a Lecturer in Psychiatry at the University of Chicago, and on the Teacher Education Faculty at the Chicago Institute for Psychoanalysis. He can be written at Francis W. Parker School, 330 W. Webster, Chicago, IL 60614.

Benjamin Garber, MD, is Director of the Barr-Harris Center for the Study of Parent Loss, Training and Supervising Analyst at the Chicago Institute for Psychoanalysis, and Associate Attending Psychiatrist at Michael Reese Hospital. He can be written at 111 N. Wabash, Chicago, IL 60602.

M. Barrie Richmond, MD, is a Training and Supervising Analyst at the Chicago Institute for Psychoanalysis, a Child and Adolescent Supervising Analyst, and Faculty Member of the Child and Adolescent Psychotherapy Program. He can be written at 449 N. Wells, Chicago, IL 60610.

Introduction

The five papers gathered in this volume are the product of two consecutive symposia on "The Care and Education of the Very Troubled Child," sponsored jointly by the Chicago Institute for Psychoanalysis and the Sonia Shankman Orthogenic School of the University of Chicago. The theme evolved out of our concern regarding the frequent misconception that a psychoanalytic perspective in the treatment of children, especially those in residential treatment, means a disregard for the parents of those children. Our conviction is quite the contrary. We believe that without the cooperation and support of the parents, therapy, including milieu therapy, is doomed. At the same time we recognize that it is very inviting for any empathic child therapist, teacher or child care worker to be critical of those parents. Thus, one of the most difficult tasks of the professional working with children is to maintain an empathic stance toward both child and parent. The psychoanalyst, with the professional tools of self analysis, is in an excellent position to understand and provide insight into the means of achieving this dual stance. These papers address areas that put greatest stress on the maintenance of this all important parental alliance: areas that are both external and internal. The application of the principles expressed to broader situations is sometimes left to the reader and sometimes, particularly in the concluding paper, spelled out.

Dr. Bleiberg's paper opens the volume with a presentation of a theoretical understanding of narcissistic personality disorder, one of the most common of the severe diagnostic categories in childhood and adolescents. We put this at the beginning to provide a view from within of some of the children about whose parents we write. In his presentation he integrates findings from infant research with a developmental perspective. His formulation leads to an understanding of the necessary components of treatment. It further permits a clear statement of the emotional conditions that, from this point of view, parents need to provide to enable a youngster to maintain treatment gains after leaving residential placement.

Dr. Childress then introduces the issue of the therapist's feelings about parents. He suggests a model of a therapeutic point of view towards parents as being well-intentioned toward their child. He suggests that when a therapist's feelings deviate from this view in either positive or negative direction (seeing the parent either as abusive or super-parent) it is time to take a self-check on one's own irrational reactions. One might, otherwise, lose the ability to, for example, help the parents to provide the kind of conditions described by Dr. Bleiberg as necessary to maintain therapeutic gains.

Dr. Childress goes on to discuss certain situations that are most conducive to losing therapeutic balance. Of particular interest is the area of child abuse, where the clarity of what actually is abuse is much murkier than we would like to believe and the best interest of the child less clear than we would like it to be.

Dr. Garber discusses in elucidating detail the problems encountered by the therapist in maintaining a constructive alliance with the parents of children who have suffered parent loss. From extensive experience at the Barr-Harris Center for parent loss, he explores and contrasts issues that arise in dealing with parents of children who have suffered loss from parental death with those that arise in dealing with children of divorce. The very different kinds of feelings that are evoked toward parents in these circumstances are clearly set out, thus detailing the pitfalls that lie in the way of a beneficial alliance.

In his paper on "Countertransference Problems with Severely Disturbed Parents," Dr. Richmond presents a theoretical framework that helps us to understand the familiar problems that all of us have had in dealing with very difficult parents of very difficult children. In open and lucid examples he documents reactions from his own experience that have led to certain actions and decisions (such as not engaging a patient for treatment) that he might have handled differently had he, at the time, greater self-awareness. Though his experience is from private practice, those of us who deal with very disturbed youngsters in all settings know how difficult, but vital, it is to cope with our own reactions to the actions and reactions of parents of very disturbed children.

Dr. Frank concludes the volume with a sensitive discussion of the multitude of factors that come into play in dealing with a disturbed youngster in a school setting. He makes clear that the setting he describes is a privileged (though not "therapeutic") one. The issues that he focuses on, however, are existent in any school setting. He reflects on the importance of understanding and considering the feelings and vulnerabilities of all involved: staff, parents, therapists and administrator. His paper is a compelling explication of how principles and insights developed in some limited settings can be usefully applied in a broader context.

Jacquelyn Seevak Sanders, PhD
Barry L. Childress, MD

The Yogi and the Commissar: Integrating Individual and Family Approaches in the Treatment of Narcissistic Children and Adolescents

Efrain Bleiberg, MD

Over the past two decades, infancy studies (Sameroff and Emde, 1989; Stern, 1985) have produced an increasingly clear and coherent picture of the unfolding and structuring of infants' and young children's subjective experience and intrapsychic reality. Such studies offer a rich opportunity to enhance our understanding of the development and pathogenesis of the severe personality disorders. In the first part of this, I will examine the implications of a developmental perspective to the conceptualization of a treatment approach for children and adolescents with a narcissistic personality disorder. In the second part, I will present a detailed clinical example to flesh out how individual and family approaches are integrated.

In particular, research has documented the biases, preferences, and predispositions built into the human brain; the motivational systems giving direction to development and to the organization of experience; and the tools for information processing, memory, perception, affect, and arousal regulation that become available to children to construct their intrapsychic world. Thus, developmental research provides a window through which to peer into the processes that lead to the structuring of particular configurations of experience and of specific coping and defensive strategies. When these psychological configurations are rigidly maintained, regardless of their maladaptive consequences, we are squarely in the domain of the personality disorders.

A brief discussion of some selected aspects of development is of relevance to support the clinical and conceptual premises of this paper.

MOTIVATIONAL SYSTEM, INTERNAL REPRESENTATIONAL MODELS, NARCISSISTIC REGULATION

Although the views emerging from infancy research support a number of psychoanalytic ideas about early development, they also challenge many assumptions held by psychoanalysts about the nature and content of the infant's psychic life. Freud's motivational theory has come under scrutiny and criticism. Developmental investigators' (Emde, 1989) account of the basic motivational systems giving direction to behavior differs sharply from Freud's. Freud, as is well known, identified the sexual and aggressive drives as *the* fundamental motivational forces, producing a build-up of tension and generating a psychologically preemptory need to discharge such tension. Developmental studies support instead the existence of an array of basic motivational systems present at birth, some of which are tension-*seeking* rather than directed at tension-reduction. Arguably, motivational systems other than sexuality and aggression play prominent–perhaps more prominent–roles in the early organization of an infant's subjective world.

Two motivational systems stand out as pivotal in the development of narcissistic regulation. Infancy research amply supports Fairbairn's (1952) seminal contention of the primacy of the human craving for sustaining connections with others. As Bowlby (1969) noted, given human beings' helplessness at birth, survival is best guaranteed–thus providing an advantage likely to be selected out by the evolutionary process–by the capacity to seek closeness and evoke protection from caretakers. The evolutionary advantage of a capacity for relatedness may explain the built-in motivation for social fittedness. As Stern (1985) mentioned, neonates are prepro-grammed to recognize people, to prefer and to seek out human stimulation, and to develop the behavioral repertoire of attachment. Thus it appears highly unlikely that the pairing of human beings for the gratification of presumably more basic biological needs is a precondition to the child's interest in relating to other humans. We are, as Greenberg and Mitchell (1983) explain, essentially drawn to relate, intrinsically gratified by relationships, and endowed with a brain inherently wired to generate, organize, and pattern psychologi-cal experience in a human, interpersonal context.

This motivational tendency correlates with a specific affective disposition. Distress escalating to overwhelming anxiety and organ-ismic vulnerability follows disruption of the infant's attachments (Bowlby, 1969, 1973; Spitz, 1965). Kandel (1983) points out that the fight and flight system built into the human brain appears ready to activate a response of anger, anxiety, and hyperarousal–the or-ganismic readiness to fight or flee–following the absence of caretak-ers. Other humans, on the other hand, claims Kandel, evoke a ready-to-be activated signal of safety, which down-regulates the fight and flight system. Thus, affective responses of anxiety and hyperarousal or safety and relaxation provide additional incentives and disincentives to channel infant behavior in the direction of establishing connections with others.

Infancy research also strongly supports the existence of a power-ful built-in predisposition toward achieving mastery and creating organization. As Emde (1989) remarks, the infant comes into the world "with biologically prepared active propensities and with organized capacities for self-regulation" (p. 35). Stern (1985) noted an innate tendency to put together in one's mind what goes together in reality, as well as a corresponding affective response of distress when organization cannot be created, or when the anticipated match between a mental schema of reality and reality itself is disrupted. Stern (1985), for example, cites studies demonstrating that if a mother's face is shown to a three-month-old infant on a television screen but her voice is delayed by a few hundred milliseconds, the infant detects the discrepancy in synchrony and is disturbed by it.

The distressing consequences of a disruption in experiential co-herence were well described in Freud's early writings. In *Studies on*

Hysteria (1893-95/1955), Freud and Breuer compared hysteria with the traumatic neurosis. In both instances, they claimed, an event had become pathogenic because it could not be integrated into the dominant mass of ideas (the psychic organization that Freud subsequently designated as the ego). Thus, the experience in question could not be processed through the normal psychological mechanisms and instead persisted, unmetabolized, seeking expression through somatic channels.

Almost 30 years later, in *Inhibition, Symptoms and Anxiety* (1920/1955), Freud conceptualized trauma as the experience of being overwhelmed by an adaptive demand that renders the ego passive, helpless, and unable to anticipate, cope, integrate, and retain a sense of control. According to Freud, the essence and meaning of the traumatic situation consists of "the subject's estimation of his own strength compared to the magnitude of the danger and his admission of helplessness" (Freud 1920, p. 166). As a corollary, Freud described the ego's tendency to attempt a turnaround of such passivity and helplessness in an effort to gain (or regain) a measure of activity and mastery. Freud believed that this tendency was critical to advancing the individual's most basic narcissistic pursuits, that is, the capacity for self-preservation.

Freud's ideas provide a framework for conceptualizing the phenomena of narcissistic vulnerability and narcissistic regulation. In contrast, however, to the opposition Freud (1915, 1917) postulated between narcissism and object relatedness, developmental studies point to an intertwining of these two motivational systems. In Greenberg and Mitchell's (1983) formulation, human beings are both self-regulating and field regulating. We are, say Greenberg and Mitchell, fundamentally concerned with both the efforts to create and maintain coherence, mastery and organization *and* with the efforts to create and maintain connections with others.

More to the point, efforts to gain mastery, reduce helplessness, and achieve experiential coherence coalesce in normal development with the pursuit of relationships in a mutually reinforcing process. Sander (1975) and Ainsworth and Bell (1974) make the point that the infant's competence is contingent on the presence of alert and responsive caregivers. To achieve a sense of mastery and produce a state of experiential coherence–and turn around their experience of passivity and helplessness brought about by adaptive demands (whether from within or from without) only by signaling distress and evoking attuned responses from their caretakers. The appropriate response, for example, to a signal of hunger, transforms the infant's internal state from that of hunger–and helplessness in the face of it–to that of satiation and a regained sense of mastery.

Such transactional sequences certainly permit the restoration of physiological homeostasis and reinforce the attachment system. They also provide the template for mental schemas of those episodes. Stern (1985) describes how the infant's abstraction of the common or invariant features of those transactional episodes leads to the construction of representations of interactions generalized (RIGs) which are subsequently organized into internal working models or internal representations of the self in relation to others. These internal representational models (IRMs) provide a prototype for the sense of self as competent and worthy, and of others as responsive. Not surprisingly, disturbances of narcissistic regulation invariably involve concerns about being ignored or not given attention, often coupled with doubts about the ability to have an impact on or to evoke responses from others.

Given this built-in motivational push toward self-regulation and object relationships, infants will almost inevitably–as soon as memory and representational capacities permit–construct IRMs both to guide their search for human connections more effectively and to anticipate reality's demands. While initially these IRMs serve to anticipate reality–and signal distress to others when there is a failure of "matching" between IRMs and external reality–as infants' competences grow they begin to utilize their IRMs to organize future interactions. Sroufe (1989) describes three- and four-year-old children attempting to break into a preschool dance at the Minnesota Preschool Project. Children assessed at age one as anxiously attached are more likely to be rebuffed when trying to break in. Following a rebuff, these children more commonly sulk and crawl to a corner. Children assessed as securely attached at age one are less likely to evoke rejection. Even when rebuffed, however, these children will typically continue trying until they break into the group. They exhibit far less evidence of feeling rejected. Instead, they persist until they evoke an interpersonal response that matches their internal model: they are worthy and effective and others are responsive.

In normal development, the tendency to utilize intrapsychic models to organize interpersonal reality is modulated by a corresponding openness of the intrapsychic world to be modified by interpersonal influences. This openness is illustrated by the phenomenon of social referencing (Campos and Sternberg, 1981; Hornik and Gunnar, 1988). When infants are confronted with a novel or uncertain situation, that is, a situation from which they lack an internal model, they seek to resolve the uncertainty by obtaining emotional clues from a caretaker. If the caretaker's face signals encouragement, they explore with pleasure. If, however, the caretaker's face betrays anxiety, they become inhibited and distressed. Thus, children are still able to attempt a representational match but mediated by information provided by the caretakers.

ACTUAL SELF, IDEAL SELF, AND NARCISSISTIC REGULATION

The growing development of categorical thinking and symbolic capacity during the second half of the second year of life provides children with an extraordinary new tool for achieving mastery, control, and experiential coherence (i.e., narcissistic well being).

Children become increasingly capable of creating a mental representation, which Joffe and Sandler (1967) call the "ideal self." This ideal self is in the shape of a self-representation associated with a sense of safety, competence, and satisfaction. The ideal self conjures up the experience of mastery, control, experiential integration, and optimal ability to meet adaptive demands. Such an "ideal self" also transacts optimally with available and responsive others.

What are the building blocks of this mental representation? According to Jaffe and Sandler, the ideal self is a composite of: (a) memories of actual experiences of pleasure, mastery, satisfaction, and competence (with particular emphasis on memories of the infant's successful evocation of caretakers' responses that lead to a restored sense of narcissistic well-being); (b) fantasies about such experiences (which become increasingly more elaborated symbolically and more available to serve defensive purposes); and (c) the models provided by important people who are loved, feared, or admired.

An example of this representational composite is found in the following vignette: a two-and-a-half-year-old boy protests loudly when his parents, both busy professionals, leave on certain evenings to attend a professional event. The parents, in attempts to comfort the child that are as driven by guilt as by empathy, tell him, "We have to go to a meeting, dear, but when you wake up, we will be back." A few weeks later, the boy is happily riding up and down the driveway on his brand new tricycle. "I'm going to a meeting," he proudly announces to his father. Rather sheepishly the father replies, "Great, Johnny, have fun." The father's endorsement, however, only elicits the child's scorn. "No, no, Daddy. . .," the child chides the father with exasperation, "Cry!" When the chastised father finally "gets it" and "weeps" in distress, the child triumphantly says, "It's okay, daddy, when you wake up, I'll be back."

This vignette illustrates the use of a model as a blueprint, a road map guiding the child's efforts to reverse states of helplessness and passivity. He is no longer the one being left but instead is the one leaving. Rather than be the recipient of the comforting, he is the one attempting to soothe. The mental representation of the object provides an internal model to "match" or approximate.

According to Joffe and Sandler (1967), narcissistic vulnerability results from the mismatch or incongruence between the ideal self and the actual self, which is the conscious and unconscious sense individuals have of their characteristics, capacities, and ability to respond to adaptive demands. The tendency toward experiential congruity now encompasses both external reality and the internal model of the ideal self.

Narcissistic vulnerability refers to a painful state of self-appraisal whose affective correlate is the feeling of shame. The prototypical affect of narcissistic vulnerability, shame reflects the sense of deflation accompanying the inability to measure up to an ideal. Narcissistic well-being or self-esteem, on the other hand, results from the successful shaping of the actual after the ideal self. Affects, as Emde (1989) has pointed out, promote the organization of experience by providing a system of incentives and disincentives for functioning both on an internal psychological level and on a social interactive context. Expression of affects also serves as a social signal that evokes responses from others.

In continuity with the phenomenon of social referencing, the efforts to match the ideal self require interpersonal validation. Parental pride and pleasure in the child's approximation of an ideal–which in part reflects the parent's own ideals–promotes the child's identificatory efforts while also bringing children and parents closer together. Thus, throughout development, narcissistic regulation and object relations potentiate each other in a context where intrapsychic models and interpersonal context are constantly shaping, modifying, and reinforcing one another.

To appreciate the role of narcissistic regulation in development, one need only examine the transition from a dyadic world to the triangular world of the Oedipal complex. The child's representational capacities during the second year facilitate achievement of a core gender identity. This aspect of the actual self is built around the organization of inner sensation; the perception of one's own and other people's genitals; and the multiple verbal and nonverbal messages, given consciously and unconsciously, that convey the family's assignment to the child of a given gender (male or female) (Stoller 1975).

Such internal constructs serve as a guide in seeking "self-like" objects, that is, the same-sex parents (Tyson 1983) to match not only in their behavior and attitudes but also in their subjective experience and intrapsychic world (Ogden 1989). In identifying with the same-sex parent, children gain a beacon that orients them in their journey of discovery during the second year of life. In their efforts to gain greater mastery and coherence, children identify with the same-sex parent as a preferential mechanism of narcissistic regulation. Children, while identifying with the same-sex parent, are also likely to attempt to match that parent's intrapsychic world, including object choices and sexual preferences, a process that powerfully pushes children toward triadic relationships (Ogden, 1989).

In order for such identification to be beneficial, it must meet these criteria from the standpoint of narcissistic regulation:

a. The model of the ideal self must be "reachable" by the child, using actual and potential capabilities and real attributes. The ideal self functions as the child's proximal area of development (Stern, 1985), that is, it serves as a preview of the person the child is about to become. The same-sex parent acquires such a privileged position in the child's ideal self because–and only when–it provides a "reachable" ideal.

b. The successful identification with the ideal results in self-esteem *and* interpersonal validation. The same sex parent is an effective model when experienced by the child as worthy and effective. Equally important is the other parent's response to the same-sex parent and to the child's attempts to "become" the same-sex parent. Parental pride and pleasure in the child's identificatory efforts with the same sex parents greatly enhance the narcissistic value of the identificatory process.

Every step in development–from maturational change to new psychosocial demands–renews the likelihood of narcissistic vulnerability. Narcissistic regulation is not "settled" in a particular developmental stage but instead provides one of the fundamental engines of growth throughout life. The ideal self–open to interpersonal influences–is constantly reshaped to function as an effective guide for reversing states of helplessness and the lack of experiential coherence. Using the ideal self as a map in the journey through life permits us to reshape our self-representation–our actual self–based on our identifications. The ideal self becomes a blueprint for finding new solutions to life's dilemmas, exploring different ways of being in the world and relating to others, and attempting behaviors and attitudes that promise greater mastery, more effective coping, and increased pleasure and adaptation.

Kernberg (1966) has described the progressive depersonification and abstraction of the ideal self as evolving toward the end of adolescence into a direction-giving psychological system of goals and ideals: the ego ideal. Although the ego ideal remains "open" to interpersonal influences, this intrapsychic system tends to acquire some degree of autonomy from external validation and reinforcement. A 2-year-old, for example, who has been told repeatedly that his favorite snack is only available after dinner may experience an acute longing for the special succor that only that morsel can bring. As a result, the child attempts–unsuccessfully–to seduce his mother into breaking the family rule. When mother is unmoved by the child's charms, he himself ends the exchange by loudly declaring, "Johnny, you cannot have fruit bars before dinner time!"

This exchange illustrates the principles involved in internalizing parental functions and identifying with the models contained in the ideal self. Faced with clear and consistent limits, the children will tend to turn around the experience of being the passive recipients of parental limits. They gain a measure of activity by modeling themselves after the limit-setting parent. Eventually, no loud declaration will have to come to the child's ears–even one produced by the child himself. A silent psychological process will have replaced it. By the end of adolescence, abstract principles and values–of self-restraint, healthy habits, etc., will replace the internal representation of a parent admonishing the child to wait until after dinner to indulge his cravings.

PATHOLOGICAL NARCISSISTIC REGULATION

Some degree of dysfunction in narcissistic regulation is present in all forms of psychopathology. The pathology disrupts the organizing capacities and abilities that people use to bring coherence to their experience. The more specific narcissistic disorders (i.e., the narcissistic personality disorder) present a particular distortion of the development and the organization of subjective experience.

Children in the process of crystallizing a narcissistic personality exhibit extremely rigid coping mechanisms that involve reliance on an omnipotent sense of self, refusal to acknowledge personal failures, projection of disowned self-experiences onto others, and demands for public affirmation of their power.

Such children clearly tend, even before their school-age years, to replace ongoing efforts to approximate a constantly maturing ideal self with a defensively derived fantasy: they develop their sense of self around an illusion of power, control, perfection, mastery, and invulnerability. The ideal self no longer functions as a blueprint to guide identificatory efforts but instead is an illusory basis for the sense of self.

They also rigidly persist in disowning, dissociating, and denying any experiences in which the self fails to measure up to the ideal. Experiences of helplessness, vulnerability, longing for others, envy, pain, or sadness, in particular, are experienced as "not me." A rigid, discontinuity of subjective experience, held onto desperately, in the face of all challenges and demands, is a hallmark of all developing personality disorders.

As part of their ongoing efforts to "rid" themselves of their rejected and dissociated self-experiences, they project them onto and attempt to evoke them in, others. Thus, other people are held in contempt or may be perceived as worthless, weak, and incompetent. Significant adults are rarely seen as reliable protectors, limit-setters, sources of support, or interpreters of reality. Instead, people are mere tools to be manipulated or objects from which to extract gratification.

They also often make angry or manipulative demands to extract from others the needed confirmation of their power, magnificence, control, or omnipotence. The narcissistic individual's insistence that the real world matches and supports a rigidly held intrapsychic configuration is another hallmark of a developing personality disorder. Yet no matter how much confirmation of omnipotence is received, the person is continually haunted by the specter of shame, the ever-present threat that any rejected vulnerability will be uncovered, paving the way for vicious attacks and humiliation.

Clinical observations of narcissistic youngsters appear to support Kernberg's (1975) notion that the development of these children is not arrested in an earlier form of narcissistic regulation but rather is becoming organized in an inflexible and distorted fashion. Narcissistic children's demands for control (whether hidden or overt), are excessive and can never be fulfilled. These children, who are unable to feel gratitude, become used to giving orders and setting the tone of the household from a remarkably young age. As Noshpitz (1983) points out, they insist on having their own way–and their parents are unable to manage them. They struggle with all their might to be the center of everyone's attention and, when frustrated, fly into a towering rage.

Their inability to expose their vulnerabilities also interferes with their schoolwork. Unable to acknowledge their limitations and accept help from their teachers, they adopt instead the stance of refusing to work rather than admitting their shortcomings. Their language may be precocious and impressive, prompting teachers to harbor expectations of academic achievement. But their verbal cleverness often expresses basically empty intellectualizations and word play. Tall tales and lies cover a limited capacity for sustained attention and difficulty with solving problems in reality. Language becomes a tool for exhibitionism and manipulation, a defense against shame, envy, and vulnerability, and a weapon to control, intimidate, and keep people at a distance.

Different developmental paths lead to these distortions in narcissistic regulation. P. Kernberg (1989) described several groups of children at particular risk for developing a narcissistic personality: children of narcissistic parents, adopted children, abused children, overindulged or wealthy children, children of divorce, and children who had lost a parent through death. Clearly, these diverse sets of developmental circumstances are unlikely to result in a homogeneous condition. Instead, several subtypes of narcissistic pathology can be distinguished in which one or more of the key elements of the narcissistic organization of experience (e.g., omnipotence, dissociation of vulnerability, control of others) is more or less emphasized.

Some of these children experienced the extreme selectivity of attunement well described by Rinsley (1989). These children evoke parental response, validation, love and pride with their precocious skills and exhibitionistic display of talents, charm, beauty, or intelligence. Parental responses are tuned to those aspects of the child that best approximate the parent's ideal self. Thus, the child's "performance" regulates parental self-esteem. On the other hand, those aspects of the child that fail to match the parent's ideal self are ignored, rejected, or ridiculed.

Other narcissistic children were pushed by the circumstances of their life to a premature closure of dependency and reliance in self-nurturing capacity. Abuse and neglect, unbearable helplessness, the inability to achieve real mastery lead resourceful youngsters to numbness, that is, the dissociation of passivity, pain and vulnerability, and the replacement of the efforts to gain real mastery from an illusion of perfection or omnipotence (Bleiberg, 1988).

TREATMENT APPROACHES:
A REPRESENTATIONAL MISMATCH

In *The Yogi and the Commissar*, Arthur Koestler described two opposing views of how to change reality. The yogi's vision is based on the notion that only internal transformations will lead to a change in reality. The commissar's view is predicated on the conviction that the only route to internal change is through achieving first a transformation of external reality.

Faced with the intimidating and deflating clinical challenge presented by narcissistic youngsters, treaters turn to yogis and commissars in search of guidance. The basic premise of this paper is that the effective treatment of narcissistic children and adolescents requires the careful integration of approaches aimed at achieving intrapsychic changes with interventions designed to facilitate changes in children's interpersonal context.

Clinical experience suggests that meaningful therapeutic engagement–let alone enduring changes–is unlikely unless there is a movement in the child's interpersonal world in a direction that creates what Horowitz (1987, 1988) calls a "representational mismatch." In Horowitz's formulation, a representational mismatch is produced when reality challenges or contradicts the expectations generated by an internal representational model. In the case of narcissistic children, a representational mismatch is created when caretakers and treaters become more competent generally, more effective and consistent limit-setters, more capable of introducing generational boundaries, and more invested in extricating narcissistic children from the special roles they often play within the family detouring one parent's hostility against the other; holding the parent's marriage together; maintaining parents' self-esteem; or preventing parental suicide. In the absence of such representational mismatch, even powerful yogis are unable to counter the pathological reinforcement provided by a "matching" reality.

From a clinical standpoint, the crucial considerations in deciding between an inpatient or residential setting, on the one hand, or an outpatient or community-based plan, on the other, are: (a) the capacity of the youngster's parents to move in the direction of competence, effective limit-setting, and generational boundaries; (b) the availability of community resources and services that can be mobilized to support parental competence; and (c) the extent of the youngster's need for containment, support, and structure. Narcissistic children respond to changes in their interpersonal environment with desperate and sometimes destructive efforts to recreate a context characterized by caretakers' ineptitude, inconsistency, and unreliability. In short, a representational mismatch generates anxiety which, in turn, mobilizes an intensification of narcissistic children's pathological defenses and interpersonal maneuvers designed to reestablish a reality supportive of their intrapsychic organization. Such maneuvers can be so destructive that effective containment surpasses the "holding" (Winnicott, 1965) ability of even well functioning families. Day treatment programs or residential treatment should be considered for these youngsters. Treatment in specialized residential treatment centers or hospitals is indicated for children with substantial borderline and/or antisocial comorbidity as well as those presenting intricate combinations of narcissistic personality with learning disabilities, ADHD, substance abuse and/or mood disorders.

Whether the treatment is conducted in an inpatient or outpatient setting, treaters can anticipate an onslaught of blatant or subtle efforts from both the narcissistic child and the parents to reestablish patterns of relationships that, while painful and maladaptive, were often lifesaving and provided a measure of safety and predictability. The critical step in the beginning phase of treatment is to establish the beginning of a therapeutic alliance between parents and treaters. Individual psychotherapy should begin only *after* parents and clinicians share an understanding of the nature of the child's difficulties and an agreement regarding the therapeutic steps needed to address those difficulties.

From a family systems perspective, the diagnostic formulation provides treaters and parents with an intellectual common ground. The family therapy literature has long documented the importance of presenting diagnostic formulations that (a) provide the parents with a historical, multigenerational context against which to look at the development of dysfunctional patterns of interaction in the family; (b) avoid siding with one parent against the other or exacerbate the parent's guilt, shame, or sense of incompetence; (c) highlight the child's part in maintaining and reinforcing dysfunctional patterns of interaction in the family every bit as much as the role of dysfunctional interactions in maintaining and reinforcing the child's psychopathology; (d) define the problems in terms of difficulties to be addressed by changes in the way people interact with one another.

Excluding the narcissistic child from the sessions designed to share a formulation and develop a treatment alliance with the parents conveys a powerful message: the adults are in charge. This message begins the process of creating a mismatch between the child's expectations and external reality.

INDIVIDUAL PSYCHOTHERAPY
AND FAMILY TREATMENT

The beginning of a representational mismatch–whether on an outpatient or an inpatient setting–allows the individual psychotherapist to focus on creating a therapeutic context in which an alliance can emerge, that is, the development in the patients of the notion that collaborative activity with the therapist is possible, safe, and potentially helpful.

Achieving such sense of collaboration is, of course, easier said than done. Therapists typically contend with ruthless tyranny, aloofness, suspiciousness, demands for control, or elaborate showmanship. Filled with bravado and pretentions of self-sufficiency, narcissistic youngsters are often bent on demeaning the therapist. They may, however, appear grateful and seemingly compliant, brimming with intellectual insights or seductively communicating their admiration for the therapists. These initial maneuvers provide a window into the subjective experience and characteristic defenses of narcissistic children. They are also the source of the greatest obstacle to therapeutic engagement: the therapist's countertransference.

Narcissistic children's efforts to "rid" themselves of pain, helplessness, and vulnerability and evoke responses supportive of their intrapsychic organization elicits: dread of the sessions; need to subjugate and sadistically retaliate against the patient; desires to show who "really is in charge"; feelings of impotence, helplessness, and masochistic surrender; secret admiration of the patient's smooth manipulativeness and toughness; erotic feelings, and the gratified sense of being the special savior of gifted but misunderstood children. The therapist's own responses provide a greater appreciation of the pressures parents are subjected to.

Initial psychotherapeutic interventions should focus simply on clarifying the patient's subjective experience ("Let me see if I understand what you are saying") while avoiding prematurely interpreting the youngster's envy, sadness, vulnerability, or rage, and the related defenses of grandiosity, dissociation, denial, and projective identification. The therapeutic intent is to facilitate the establishment of a beachhead, an area of the child's experience that can be safely shared with the therapist.

Premature confrontation of the patient's defenses or narcissistic vulnerability before this beachhead is established only exacerbates the need for distance, control, or devaluation. On the other hand, interventions that help the youngsters save face–protecting them from unbearable narcissistic vulnerability–can pave the way for a therapeutic alliance. "Face-saving" interventions include assisting patients in maintaining a sense of control when confronted with the representational mismatch introduced by adult's competence and limit-setting. The therapeutic challenge is to maintain a balance between fostering more adaptive solutions to reality's demands, maintaining a semblance of control, and keeping anxiety and narcissistic vulnerability within manageable limits.

Children's readiness to enter the middle phase of therapy is signaled by two indicators: the obvious appearance of anxiety and the beginning of a therapeutic alliance. Anxiety is generated largely by the representational mismatch created by the adult's limits and competence. To some degree, however, anxiety also can be traced to the children's own wishes for closeness with their therapists and the dawning conviction (fraught with uncertainty and fears of being subjugated, destroyed, or humiliated) that hope and help can be derived from therapeutic relationships.

Only rarely can these youngsters openly acknowledge their attachment to their therapists. More commonly, children can demonstrate some embryonic collaboration in the form of sharing experiences with the therapists or in using their treaters to find face-saving solutions to the adults' "conspiracy" to deprive them of their usual coping mechanisms.

The presence of some form of collaborative relationships allows therapists to gently encourage their patients to consider an expansion in the range of "shareable" experiences: narcissistic youngsters are invited to share their experiences of vulnerability, depression, pain, helplessness, and dependency.

Only at this point can therapists attempt to systematically confront children's characteristic defenses and begin the exploration of the motives and functions of those defenses. However, as children face their vulnerability, pain, and depression, they are filled with stark panic.

Not surprisingly, a heightened reliance on old defensive mechanisms becomes apparent, i.e., efforts to control, devalue, intimidate, manipulate, or seduce the therapists, rejection of help, running away, abuse of drugs, and intensified antisocial behavior outside of the sessions, or attempts to pit parents and therapists against each other.

Joe, a 13-year-old borderline narcissistic boy, had been subjected to brutal physical and sexual abuse by an alcoholic father, while his mother pursued her theatrical career. Almost in spite of himself he began to feel more comfortable with me, even to look forward to the sessions. Yet, desires for closeness were almost unbearable for him. Thus, he began to carefully look for "mistakes"–interrupting him or "invading" his space while walking–which triggered hateful barrages. He let me know of his plans to run away from the hospital, find out my house's location–"I have good sources, you know"–so he could set it on fire after raping my wife and murdering my children with slow, intravenous injections of cocaine. He would spare my life, but only to ensure that I would suffer the devastation of the loss of everything I hold dear.

Joe's tirade spoke volumes of what closeness meant to him: a painful, destructive invasion of his house-fortress, a rape, a painful penetration of his body and bloodstream that could evoke burning, devastating feelings leading to total collapse; the envy of my possessions and my relationships and the associated rage at his own deprivation and abuse; the wish to eliminate all possible rivals for my love but also the desire to leave me as deprived, lonely, and needy as him.

Obviously, such outbursts evoke rather intense countertransferential responses in the treaters. Interestingly, while attempting to weather the storm of Joe's vindictive rage, I felt neither threatened nor cut off from him. I wondered if he wished to provoke me yet remain connected to me, all the while denying any attachment. He did not love me, he seemed to tell me. In fact, he hated me. I was a pedantic, know-it-all, rich shrink who could not possibly understand someone steeled by a life in the mean streets of the big city.

Sensing his desire to maintain a relationship while overtly disowning it, I commented on the meanness and cruelty of his imagery. Where did that come from? He looked at me with a mix of contempt and amusement and proceeded to describe, in a wildly exaggerated fashion, the toughness of his neighborhood and its brutal gang wars. He was sure that my wimpy, nerdy self had been shielded from such roughness.

Together with contempt and devaluation, I sensed an inviting, playful teasingness in Joe's account of his gang escapades. In effect, he had grown up in the far more sedate environment of an upper middle class community in New England. His interest and knowledge of gangs had mostly been acquired through extensive reading on the subject. Prior to his outburst he had brought to the sessions magazines and tapes glorifying the Bloods, the Latin Kings, and other equally unsavory characters.

I picked up (perhaps with more hope than conviction) on the implied teasing and replied with an even more fantastic account of my own heroic battles as a gang kingpin—a secret identity hidden behind my deceptively mild appearance.

He seemed to enjoy this gambit and over the next few sessions we engaged in a good deal of increasingly more good natured bantering. Only after we had reestablished our relationship at a distance he could more readily tolerate did I bring back to his attention the rage he had experienced and the abuse he had inflicted upon me.

This vignette illustrates how these youngsters often require a transitional area of relatedness akin to Winnicott's (1953) transitional experience. In this transitional, as-if area (often jointly created by patient and therapist) standing between fantasy and reality, patients can both own and disown their rejected feelings and experiences and test out the therapist's attunement, respect, and responsiveness to the vulnerable aspects of the self.

Younger narcissistic patients often introduce, as a transitional relationship, a play theme involving an imaginary twin. The twin typically embodies the "weak," dependent, sad, helpless experiences these children find unbearable. Another version of the transitional experience, common to all children with conduct disorders, are somatic complaints. These complaints offer a way of requesting help without acknowledging it and of reconnecting with feelings of pain and inadequacy while keeping open the possibility of disowning such feelings.

Tooley's (1973) "Playing It Right" is a beautiful account of how the therapist can more closely attempt to align borderline children's play and fantasy to reality's constraints. Gradually, children are nudged to introduce small modifications in their play to better encompass the complexities, limitations, conflicts, and frustrations of reality. The transitional space of play and fantasy becomes a stage in which to try out new identifications to practice imagined solutions to life's dilemmas, to explore new ways of being in the world and relating to others, and to test behavior that promises greater mastery, more effective coping, and increased pleasure and adaptation. In the safe haven of the transitional sphere of relatedness, therapists can safely confront children with the systematic exploration of the youngsters' pathological defenses and the motives for such defenses. Thus, in a transitional space children can be invited to consider that a whole section of their experience stands unlived, so to speak, never owned nor shared.

Therapists' acknowledgment of the utter terror children feel as they enter into a rejected, dissociated, denied aspect of their lives and relationships can prevent therapeutic stalemates and limit regression. Therapists should always point out the many advantages of *not* changing, in effect the price children would pay if they were to give up their maladaptive, but often life saving defenses. Ultimately, therapists present to their patients, implicitly or explicitly, a therapeutic "bargain": relinquishing pathological defenses and the illusion of control and safety they provide for the far more exposed and laborious process of attempting to achieve real mastery and meaningful relationships.

Such a "bargain" is unlikely to prove appealing unless a number of factors are operant in the childrens' interpersonal world. Family treatment must address the powerful coalitions often apparent between one of the parents and the symptomatic child. It is particularly imperative to extricate these children from their roles as saviors, confidants, or special partners of one of the parents (typically the other-sex parent). At the same time, opportunities should be provided to foster the relationship between children and the same-sex parents, while promoting the ability of those same-sex parents to function as models to their children (a relationship that requires the other parent's sanction).

The family therapist gives the individual psychotherapist access to a vantage point from which to assess the consequences to the family of the patient's relinquishment of symptoms and the anxieties that the child's changes may trigger in the family. Bringing the parents into the treatment serves to address a major source of resistance to treatment: an overwhelming anxiety that their growth and change will shatter the family and cause the parents to hurt one another, divorce, commit suicide, or abandon the patient.

The child's involvement in treatment, in turn, typically mobilizes parental efforts to undermine such engagement. A concerted effort is required in the family therapy sessions to both enhance parents' view of themselves as competent and to highlight that a parent's perception of the child's distress does not obviate his/her need for clear limits. Family therapy places parents in a therapeutic bind when confronting them with the child's conviction that his/her changing will be intolerable to the parents.

Increasing parent's capacity to express concern directly and give and receive support and nurturance helps address the family's feelings of exhaustion and depletion. Encouraging one or both parents to tell stories to their children of times when they felt distressed and in need of support introduces a new level of acceptability to the experience of vulnerability. It also allows for the giving and receiving of nurturance without requiring the rescue of one or another family member in indirect, provocative, or disguised fashions.

Interventions that change children's interpersonal context help bring to the fore material usefully pursued in individual psychotherapy. Themes of dependency, safety, autonomy, envy, rage, and vulnerability become available for exploration, often mixed with themes of Oedipal competition, fears of body integrity and unconscious guilt over destructive wishes. Just as important as the attunement to feelings of real pain and vulnerability is the therapists' sharing in the real joy, renewed hope, and genuine pride children experience as a result of their growth, increased competence, and comfort with their feelings.

The harbingers of termination are found both within and without the therapy process. Naturally, a sustained amelioration of symptomatic behavior is a hopeful sign. The achievement of non-delinquent peer relationships and interests is perhaps more significant than the simple absence of overt antisocial activities. Changes in family interaction and school functioning are particularly important. Children's growing ability to utilize their parents–and/or other non-delinquent adults–as sources of protection, comfort, and models of identification bodes the end of the psychotherapeutic process. When children can approach parents and teachers for help in solving problems in reality the beginning of termination is in view.

Within the therapeutic process itself, therapists recognize other clues of impending termination: children's open acknowledgment of missing the therapists during interruptions and vacations; youngsters' expressions of gratitude for help received; patients spontaneously bringing to the sessions their sense of how they utilize outside of the sessions something they learned in therapy; and perhaps the most sensitive clue, the patients bringing to the sessions their sense of loss for missed or botched opportunities and life's unfairness.

The final stage of psychotherapy offers a chance to test children's readiness to relinquish pathological defenses. Beginning to discuss with patients and parents a termination date fuels anxiety and often brings about a reactivation of symptoms in the patient and of dysfunctional interaction patterns in the parents.

Mourning the anticipated loss of the therapy and the therapist is an essential task of the termination phase. Just as important is the opportunity to work through children's and parent's disappointments: with their own shortcomings, with the adults that never measured up to their expectations, with everything they could not achieve in therapy, and with the therapists' limitations.

Regardless of the apparent regression and symptomatic reactivation, the termination phase requires a relaxation of supervision, an expression of confidence in parent's competence.

This sketchy review fails to do justice to the complexity of the therapeutic efforts designed to break the grip that anger, anxiety, and narcissistic vulnerability have fastened on the loneliness of children and the self-respect of parents.

REFERENCES

Ainsworth, M. and Bell, S. (1974). Mother-infant interaction and the development of competence. In K. Connelly and J. Bruner (Eds.), *The Growth of Competence*. New York: Academic Press.

Bleiberg, E. (1988). Developmental pathogenesis of narcissistic disorders in children. *Bulletin of the Menninger Clinic* 52, 3-15.

Bowlby, J. (1969). *Attachment*, Vol. I. New York: Basic Books.

Bowlby, J. (1973). *Separation: Anxiety and Anger*, Vol. II. New York: Basic Books.

Breuer, J. and Freud, S. (1893). Studies on Hysteria. In J. Strachey (Ed.), *The Standard Edition of the Complete Psychological Works of Sigmund Freud* Vol. II.

Campos, J. J. & Stenberg, C. (1981). Perception, appraisal, and emotion: the onset of social referencing. In M. Lamb & L. A. Sherrod (Eds.), *Infant Social Cognition*. Hillsdale, N. J.: Lawrence Erlbaum, pp. 273-314.

Emde, R. (1989). The infant's relationship experience: developmental and affective aspects. In Sameroff, A. & Emde, R. (Eds.), *Relationship Disturbances in Early Childhood*. New York: Basic Books, pp. 33-51.

Fairbairn, W. R. D. (1952). *An Object Relations Theory of the Personality*. New York: Basic Books.

Freud, S. (1926). Inhibitions, symptoms and anxiety. In J. Strachey (Ed.) *The Standard Edition*, Vol. XX. London: Hogarth Press, 1957, 77-178.

Hornik, R. & Gunnar, M. R. (1988). A descriptive analysis of infant social referencing. *Child Development* 59, 626-634.

Horowitz, M. J. (1987). *States of Mind: Configurational Analysis of Individual Personality*. New York: Plenum Press.

Horowitz, M. J. (1988). *Introduction to Psychodynamics*. New York: Basic Books.

Joffe, N. G. & Sandler, J. (1967). Some conceptual problems involved in the consideration of disorders of narcissism. *Journal of Child Psychotherapy* 2(1), 56-66.

Kandel, E. (1983). From metapsychology to molecular biology: explorations into the nature of anxiety. *American Journal of Psychiatry* Vol. 140:1277-1293.

Kernberg, O. (1966). *Object Relations Theory and Clinical Psychoanalysis.* New York: J. Aronson.

Kernberg, O. (1975). *Borderline Conditions and Pathological Narcissism.* New York: J. Aronson.

Kernberg, P. (1989). Narcissistic personality disorder in childhood. In Otto F. Kernberg (Ed.), *The Psychiatric Clinics of North America* Vol. 12, No. 3, pp. 671-694.

Koestler, A. (1975) *The Yogi and the Commissar.* McMillan Publish.

Noshpitz, J. (1984). Narcissism and Aggression. *American Journal of Psychotherapy* 38, 17-34.

Ogden, T. (1989). *The Primitive Edge of Experience.* New York: J. Aronson.

Rinsley, D. B. (1989). Notes on the developmental pathogenesis of narcissistic personality disorders. In Otto F. Kernberg (Ed.), *Psychiatric Clinics of North America* Vol. 13, No. 3, pp. 695-707.

Sameroff, A. & Emde, R. (1989). *Relationship Disturbances in Early Childhood.* New York: Basic Books.

Sander, L. (1975). Infant and caretaking environment: investigation of conceptualization of adaptive behavior in a system of increasing complexity. In E. J. Anthony (Ed.), *Explorations in Child Psychiatry.* New York: Plenum Press.

Spitz, R. (1965). *The First Year of Life.* New York: International Universities Press.

Sroufe, L. A. (1989). Relationships, self, and individual adaptation. In Sameroff, A. & Emde, R. (Eds.), New York: Basic Books.

Stern, D. (1985). *The Interpersonal World of the Infant.* New York: Basic Books.

Stoller, R. (1975). *Sex and Gender.* New York: Science House.

Tooley K. Playing it right–a technique for the treatment of borderline children. *J Am Acad of Child Psychiat* 12:615-631, 1973.

Tyson, P. (1982). A developmental line of gender identity, gender role and choice of love object. *Journal of the American Psychoanalytic.*

Winnicott DW. *The Maturational Processes and the Facilitating Environment.* New York: Int Univ Press, 1965.

Winnicott DW. Transitional objects and transitional phenomena. *Int J Psychoanal* 34(2) 89-97, 1953.

Winnicott DW. Transitional objects and transitional phenomena. *Int J Psychoanal* 34(2) 89-97, 1953.

Thinking About Parents
and Rescuing Children

Barry L. Childress, MD

I want to talk some about parents and our ideas about them that influence our work with children. Parents can be seen as friends or foes. They can be seen as allies in their child's treatment. They can be seen as the current source of distress as in death, divorce, and abuse (they could also be seen as needing assistance in these matters). They can be seen, in reconstruction, as the original source of current symptoms.

I was recently rereading Anna Freud's 1949 paper on preadolescent children and their relationship with their parents. In this paper she discusses the family romance fantasy. The growing child views his/her parent with an increasingly realistic eye and finally says "who are these people? I must have been adopted as I dimly recall being with parents of wealth and power for a time." These parents are, of course, the omnipotent parents of early childhood. This family romance theme of deidealization of parents of the present is repeated in a more intense form in adolescence. It is here where adopted children may get derailed and imagine that it is not the omnipotent adoptive parents of childhood that they are thinking of but their biological parents instead. If this is in adolescence and the child is being difficult, the adoptive parent might also get confused and say "this can't have anything to do with me, it must come from their "real" (biological) parents." This derailment, in extreme cases, can lead to disadoption which is all too easy a legal out–and one which natural parents of adolescents might well consider if it were thought an option.

Racker, in his 1968 book on transference and countertransference in working with adult analysands, considered the phenomena both of identifying with the patient as child and of identifying with the parent of the patient as child. Those of us who work with children tend to identify with them. Actually it is very hard to see the world from that perspective. The concept of children as people with a perspective worth considering, represents a relatively recent development–most of our laws evolved from the idea of children as chattel. Even now when the law decides what is fair–it still is often fair only from the adult's point of view: e.g., a child, after living with foster parents from the ages of three months to five years can be reclaimed by biological parents through legal action.

People who have devoted themselves to work with children, however, may give parents short shrift. I think that it is hard for us all to let go of the omnipotent parents of our childhood–the parents of the family romance who could have made everything right (if my mother had done her job better, it would not have taken so long for me to have come to that realization).

Eisler constructed a base model for analytic treatment based on the concept of an ego which would ideally respond simply to the interpretation of transference and resistance. Winnicott, Gill, and Lipton have all given testimony as to the impossibility of this really happening. But with this theoretical model, we can identify any interaction which deviates from that model and try to understand its cause and its meaning–meaning to the patient in transference and meaning to the analyst in counter-transference–which is what analysis is all about.

A base model of a parent who always wants to be a good parent can similarly be constructed. The question is what interferes with the parents' doing their job well. If this is asked uncritically, parents can often be engaged in the process. Parents appreciate being treated as people–though they often don't expect it when dealing with mental health professionals about the emotional problems of their children. They expect criticism, as they are critical of themselves in their heart of hearts. Even this self blame may be a narcissistic defense against their feeling of helplessness in their efforts to influence their child's development. Parents should not take too much blame nor too much credit.

Deviation in our feeling toward the parent from benign acceptance of the parent as well-meaning, to aggravation at the parent as abusive, or to awe at the parent as super-being, requires a mental check as to what is being stimulated in our counter-transference. Sam Weiss, in a series of three papers on the technique of child analysis, highlighted the ubiquitousness of the search for the omnipotent parent. We overvalue the strength of the parent, crediting him or her with the power to cause psychopathology, and get angry at them for not parenting right. Or, as in some omnipotent battle of the Titans, we may feel that they are using their black magic to interfere with our own potential to be omnipotent curers ourselves. Our child patient may represent our child self reincarnated, doomed to imperfection because of the malevolent acts of omnipotent parents. We should be so powerful!

There are a number of situations which typically make it more difficult for us to recognize that we have lost sight of the base model of the "well intentioned parent." It can happen at any time, but some circumstances provide more fertile fields. Adolescents are difficult because they are in a stage crawling with externalizations—they are distracted and distract us with external reality. Adoption and the question of who the "real parent" is—the biological parent or the parent of childhood—is another clear example of situations that are unclear. The perspective allowed by the monitoring of transference and countertransference is hard won and not easily held. Three more situations that demand additional vigilance are death, divorce and abuse.

External reality can distract us. Treatment for the child who has lost a parent is often not immediately indicated beyond guidance to the surviving family. The focus is appropriately on externals, though hopefully the importance of personal meanings will be present in the process of such an evaluation or course of guidance. As the loss of one parent often means the loss of the second through grief and emotional unavailability, such help is likely to be prophylactic. It is at a later time when analytic intervention may become indicated that the longing for the analyst/therapist as real parent can be interpreted meaningfully as a defense.

In families where surviving parents have remarried, the conflicting areas of loyalty are similar to those of cases of divorce. The problem with divorces is that they are rarely so clear cut, or so mercifully swift, as deaths. They are more complex for the child in that the lost parent continues to exist–but with some function having been given up. Divorces can go on for years longer than the actual marriage and with more emotional intensity, albeit negative and hateful. Like with parent death, analysis is most helpful after there has been some stabilization of the child's life as represented by a truce or parenting alliance between the divorcing parents. Otherwise the ongoing trauma of parental battles may interfere with unfolding development. Such developmental interferences, as described by Nagera (1966), will be too much of a distraction and interference to the establishment of an analytic situation.

A cautious optimism about the possibility of engaging divorced parents in a therapeutic alliance which will support a child's psychotherapy seems warranted. Parents (even the designated uninvolved "bad" one) can be told that the divorce process and related legal processes understandably polarize their positions and that, fortunately, it is not necessary to find out what is really going on–of importance is only their child's reality. Their child has to be caught up in a conflict of loyalty and a struggle about their different representations of reality. The one thing that they are most likely to agree on is their wish to help their child. Parents can be invited to call at any time that they are so inclined. They must believe that the therapist is interested in what they have on their minds if there is to be any hope of managing the parental transferences which might interfere with their alliance. It can be made clear that even if direct advice won't be forthcoming there is interest in maintaining contact. Without some sense of bilateral support for a buffered area to contain the child's treatment, then treatment should be postponed while the resistances in the parents are explored. A statement from the therapist to this effect is, in itself, a strong interpretation to the parents! The attention demanded in the management of the external reality precludes true analytic work but allows significant psychotherapeutic intervention, and, if this helps to stabilize the child's position, a later analysis, if indicated, may be possible.

I had mentioned how external reality can be a distraction in these matters, but this is even more true in matters of reconstruction--when there is less than clear evidence of current abuse or when we are thinking about matters from the past. The most firm base we have for reconstructions is the actual transference material in the present and the only history that we can be fairly certain of is the actual history of the treatment.

Jeffrey Mason, a former analyst, has written a number of semi-professional, semi-popular books concerning Freud's original seduction hypothesis. Freud first postulated that neuroses were caused by actual seductions. After realizing the number of parents who would have to be seducing their children, and after fathering several children of his own, and after undertaking his own self analysis, Freud found that children had an active fantasy life which was easy to overlook. The importance of conscious and unconscious fantasy was what Freud pioneered. He never turned his back on the impact of actual seductions, as Mason charges, but, rather, he discovered the additional contribution of children's fantasy. Freud thought that inner and outer reality interacted in a complementary series in the creation of neurotic symptoms--a lot of external trauma and a little fantasy blending into a lot of fantasy and a little external reality in a continuum. The contribution of psychoanalysis was to focus on the past that was recreated in the present through the transference. Although much can be made of the importance of reconstructing truths from the past to explain current symptoms, it is not always clear how much these reconstructions are anchored in the analytic situation nor how much they actually correspond with the historical external reality. The mistakes of the seduction hypothesis can be repeated in the unsupported clinical hypotheses of other parental failures (in empathy, etc.).

It is easy to get lost in patients' descriptions of things that go on in their lives outside of the analytic office--abusive bosses, seductive women, faulty parents, and dreams of threatening monsters. Much of analytic work is in discovering how talk of bosses, women, and monsters relate to patients' reactions to their regular interaction with their analysts. There are nooks and crevices in such interactions providing justifications for earlier perceptions found now in the transference. The big red "X" of the here and now is an anchor for both patient and analyst--"X"--"you are here."

It is always easier when patients have miracle workers and ge-
niuses on their minds–that obviously refers to the analyst or something that the analyst has recently said–it is more difficult to remember that this is still transference and no more credit can be
claimed for it. Thoughts of malicious people, however–where might
they belong–surely there must "really" be an abusive boss or mon-
ster "out there" or defective parent "back there." Negative feelings that come up in sessions ought not to be routinely ascribed to
a patient's parents. Although parents surely frustrate, hurt, and
aggravate their children, that is not all they have done. Children
simply cannot have had parents who treated them only badly–it is
too easy an explanation for behavior–if only my parents had . . . fill
in the blank.

Winnicott said that, as children, we have all been hurt by our
parents but that it does no good to simply sympathize with our
patients' misfortunes. What we must do in treatment is help our
patients see how they are now the authors of the recreations of
those early traumas in the treatment and, therefore, in their current
lives.

The idea that a family can be all bad as well as the idea that
society can really replace parents and repair abused children's ails
must be carefully considered. In 1987, Dr. Albert Solnit spoke on
children, abuse, and legislated parenting alternatives at a conference
sponsored by the Juvenile Protective Association here in Chicago.
Dr. Solnit had been associated with Anna Freud and a series of
publications related to the best interest of the child. He called attention to the sweep of development in American and English social
history, referred to above, from children as possessions (chattel
similar to slaves before the Civil War) to children as entities de-
serving individual respect. There is a continued struggle of rectify-
ing the differences between the priorities of adults and children. It
is very hard to see things through the eyes of a child and so decisions are often made in fairness but it is too often fairness through
the eyes of the adult.

There is a necessary balance between families and state. The
family of the developing child must both represent society and
buffer the child from it. The importance of this autonomous family
cannot be overlooked. When a family disqualifies itself from the

protection of its children, the state must provide this guaranteed protection–but it cannot be thought of as the equivalent of what a child would experience growing up with its own family.

Solnit championed the people who worked with disadvantaged children wanting to protect them from the attacks of the press in exposing their mistakes without regard for their monumental tasks and their successes. The stress on the caseworker is phenomenal–on the front lines, in a position that is not highly esteemed, and for which there is often insufficient training. Caseworkers know that if anything bad happens, as it's bound to, they will be second guessed.

Dispositions of the children removed from their parents must be soft-hearted and tough-minded–what does a child need ideally and what is available. Time is an often unrecognized factor in the matter of dealing with a developing child. A "protective" placement can become a trauma itself, as it continues, because it cannot approach the importance of the family of origin for the developmental processes that are rampantly unfolding within the young developing child. People in the helping fields do not like to recognize that their attempts at helping can be hurtful. If a child is having difficulty, we would prefer to see it as coming from somewhere else rather than wondering if it is our help that is abusive.

There is no question that physical and sexual abuse exists. Child abuse, in all gradients, from the parents you hear screaming at their children in K Marts, to sexual seduction to brutalization and even cannibalization, most definitely exists. There remains a question as to what can be done about it. In considering such matters, we must, however, consider children's developmental stages and children's perceptions–including their attachment to a purported abuser. First, do no harm!

Despite (or because of) the intense affective reactions generated in adults when they think of an abused child, the matter of parental alliances must be considered. The importance of family must be considered–family refers to the psychological family as there are frightening chattel laws which allow biological parents to assert their rights and reclaim "their" children. Forming a parental alliance demands a great deal of work mastering the tremendous counter-transference reactions to parents we wish to dismiss.

When claims of child abuse are made in the present without clear evidence or in a reconstruction of the past, care must be taken. The impact of need on perception must be considered as was so well illustrated in the classic film *Rashomon*. This Japanese film was redone very poorly here in American under the title of *Outrage*. The original, directed in 1951 by Akira Kurosawa, takes place in the 1200's. Travelers meet in a medieval forest. A bandit kills a nobleman and rapes his wife; or did he? The same meeting is repeated as seen through the eyes of various witnesses and participants–all amazingly different. It's a matter of perspective–internal and external reality–our perceptions are distorted by often hidden needs. A simple truth is hard to come by, and this is a good representation of attempts to find out what really happened in child abuse situations. More recently the National Committee for the Prevention of Child Abuse released a 30 minute documentary titled *Child of Rage–a Story of Child Abuse*. The film was well intentioned and moving in its depiction of the impact of abuse on a six year-old girl who is treated and improves. It should promote matters of child welfare; however, a few interchanges in this film can be highlighted–not because the film was bad–but because it captures several of the areas that make working with child abuse so difficult. It also avoids the difficulty of talking about private case material and confidentiality since this material is in the public domain.

Children are usually compliant with an authority and want to be loved. These characteristics predispose them to be taken advantage of in both sexual and interview situations. In the film a girl, now 6, lost her mother when she was 12 months old. Since she was 19 months at the time of adoption and her brother was 7 months, the mother must have died around the time of the brother's birth. They were described as healthy when offered for adoption to a minister and his wife who were childless. The couple accepted the children and a few months later learned that the children had been removed from the father's home in a state of neglect, lack of food, soiled diapers, and understimulation of the boy so that he could not even roll over by himself. The parents say that this helped them understand some unspecified behaviors in the kids. Some unknown time later the girl, Beth, has a dream that a man falls on her and hurts her with a part of his body which leads the adoptive parents to suspect sexual abuse. It is hard to get a sense of the true time passage for the 4 years of this girl's life depicted in this documentary.

The film opened with Beth saying "I hurt myself the most." We then see, reportedly from tapes of actual therapy sessions, Beth talking about how hurtful she is to her brother and parents, frighteningly matter of fact. She appears to be close to her current 6 years of age–maybe 5. She talks of being abusive to her brother, especially his genitals, being abusive to family pets–sticking pins into them–and wishing to stab her parents with knives at night.

Watching this film there was no question that this child was disturbed and little question that she too had been neglected following her mother's death. All of the adults pictured were well meaning; however, the fact of her sexual abuse was not convincing–she may have been–but there were things in the presentation that were bothersome and distracting. Perhaps these were artifacts of creating a film–but if that's the case, their impact on child behavior remains to be considered in real life.

The fact that Beth is later shown as a taped performer singing in church cannot be ignored. The girl in the taped interviews with her therapist was very attentive to the therapist's face for cues, especially when she was hesitant about her answers. This was, perhaps, a vestige of the bob and weave often recorded by infant observers as very early communications between mother and infant. At times she got leading questions. There was some time leap in the presentation so that when we hear the therapist talking about the now old dream of the man falling on her, the therapist himself refers to the man as her natural father. Perhaps that had been established in an earlier therapeutic dialogue. The girl talks of the father handling her genitals but, interestingly, at the same time talks about her masturbating herself until she was raw. The therapist appears to accept the child's response that she remembers her father's actions from when she was "one year old."

At one point, when the interviewer cannot get the answers he wants, he says, "it's hard for you to remember, huh." He ignored her fragmented recollection of an event surrounding the death of some baby birds and went to what mother had said. When she comes through and seems tearful talking of upsetting things, he says, "You're doing good"–perhaps supportive and perhaps manipulative. Kids can be directed in this fashion without their conscious awareness, interviewers can direct in this fashion without their conscious awareness.

The girl is apparently temporarily removed from the adoptive home and improves in a setting where her goodness is emphasized, and she is shown feeding and caring for farm animals. Finally, she was asked twice the question, "Who did you hurt the most?" She responded emphatically "my brother" both times. A different person asks her the third time and she responds, "I hurt myself the most" which I hope you recall was the film's opening line.

I have found that it is pointless to try to second guess dynamics from a film or written case report, but I'll tell you what I was bothered by. There wasn't anything said about the mother who died, the father who was lost, or of the one child whom we can be sure was sexually abused, the brother–by Beth. Why didn't he need treatment? Perhaps 20 years ago, I saw a boy of 3 or 3 1/2 who was mutilating himself, tearing out his hair, ripping at his ears, beating himself to the point of leaving bruises, and deeply scratching his own skin. He wouldn't talk, but would only scream in despair and call himself bad. This had not happened immediately after he had been adopted but, once started, seemed accelerated by his parents' attempts to stop this awful behavior. They figured that it had to be related to his having lived with his mother for so long. She was described as a schizophrenic. He had to be hospitalized.

His parents were by profession strict disciplinarians, but nice, educated, and wanting to do the right thing and avoid doing the harmful things that others did. This was part of their expressed motivation for the adoption. They had tried to make the child behave and be good and organized and make his own bed, but he could not do the simplest thing and then would not do the simplest thing and then began to injure himself.

They paid for his hospitalization, but had already decided that they were disadopting him– an example of this all too easy process involving a small child. Often by the time parents appear with adopted children for help they have already made up their minds to rid themselves of a burden. As I have already mentioned, this is a consideration that some biologic parents might pursue if they thought that it an option. Here is an area where community education could be very helpful to adoptive families if provided before they are ready to give up.

The boy improved in the hospital–mainly through play therapy with a "bad" doll which allowed him to be first abuser and then soother; finally, he could talk about his missing beloved schizophrenic mother. A relatively non-traumatic transition from the hospital to his adoption agency was managed; there was no follow-up, but it seems likely that at that time not enough thought was given to the importance of family and the tragedy of multiple placement. The schizophrenic mother seemed a reasonable explanation for the child's behavior which distracted from the impact of well-meaning parents who were so out of synch with the here and now of that child. Similar things can occur with therapists' reconstructions of parental failures.

This kind of displacement of focus is a common problem with adopted children–especially when they get to be adolescent–and a pain–and sexual. The adoptive parents say, "You didn't get that behavior from me: you got that from your promiscuous, over sexed, over aggressive, impulsive natural parents–I disadopt thee." As I referred to earlier in talking of Anna Freud's family romance paper, most kids have some fantasy, even if fleeting, that they have been adopted and long for their real parents who are usually envisioned as rich and powerful. The problem with adopted kids is that reality confuses them–they think they are longing for their biological parents while most often they are longing for the (adoptive) parents of infancy who seemed much more rich and powerful back then. So from both parental and child perspectives there is a push to see the source of the problem or the solution from outside the family system and the self. They lose sight of the big red "X" and "you are here" notation. We can all lose sight of that.

Two more brief vignettes with this focus before closing. A baby had been taken from its mother because of her drug involvement. When the mother came to visit, the child would howl angrily, and the personnel felt that this was proof that the mother was a bad one. The mother (feeling guilty anyway) began to feel that the staff didn't like her. She thought that maybe she really was bad, and so was increasingly awkward with the staff and tense in interaction with the baby who howled even more. There was some movement to plan permanent separation of this baby from its "bad mother" even though the mother had been successfully engaged in a drug program and wanted her baby as evidenced by her participation in the visitation program. A suggestion was made that the baby's anger at the mother might, in fact be a testament to the mother's importance to the baby who was angry at having been abandoned by such a good person. The whole cycle then reversed and there appeared good staff, good mother, and good baby. The adult perspective and the child perspective.

It is not often possible to tell from a surface observation of an event what the meaning is to each individual–a la *Rashomon*. At one time in my office building new cleaning ladies were employed and began to come in to clean before I had finished my day, and at times when I might still be with patients. I tried several times to explain that they should not come in if the waiting room was unlocked and the lights were on, but there were language barriers. In the middle of an analytic hour, I heard the key in the door and saw the door open. I jumped up and saw the offender out. The analytic process was disrupted for quite a while, in spite of my attempts to understand my patient's upset in terms of the intrusion or my failure to provide a secure environment as a repetition of earlier experiences. It was only when I understood that the patient had identified with the intruder and the corresponding wishes from childhood that I understood the identification with the offender and the fantasy of being dealt with in a similar fashion.

Children respond in exactly the same way, if we are angry at the apparent intruder/abuser they will be troubled by their hidden identification with the perpetrator–even abusers from outside the family. Matters are further complicated by their egocentricity which makes them the centers of other's actions and in their mind responsible anyway. Children, also, fear being yelled at in their turn.

There are other forms of child abuse which should be noted. There are lawyers, therapists, and parents who will keep a traumatic event alive in the mind of a child for years to keep them as good testifiers. There are organizations whose evaluative techniques (separation, genital physical examination, anatomically correct doll play, and interviews) find a high percentage of sexually abused children in their evaluations. There are divorcing/divorced parents who maintain for years a more intense relationship (albeit hateful) than they ever had in their marriage. And I must include therapists who take advantage of their patients' trust for their own satisfaction, as a form of abuse of adults in therapeutic regression.

I think that the counter-transference issues concerning fantasies about omnipotent parents can be useful at any level of intervention. The omnipotent parent does not exist, except in our dim recollections, and certainly cannot be created in any existing alternatives provided by legal/social agencies. Psychotherapies, psychoanalyses, limited hospitalizations, and even limited residential treatment facilities, in my opinion, would do better to facilitate an alliance and accept (or augment) the resources of the imperfect family, rather than to try to routinely replace them. A facility such as the Orthogenic School might represent the rare setting in which disturbed children can be allowed the time and experience to be reparented by a "good enough" Institution. Even here, my understanding is that the therapeutic alliance with the actual parents is a valued feature of the program. The parents are not meant to be condemned, but, rather, the goal is the establishment of an alternate dominant internal structure for the benefit of the child rather than as condemnation of the parents.

REFERENCES

Eissler, K.R. (1953), The effect of the structure of the ego on psychoanalytic technique. *J. Amer. Psychoanal. Assn.*, 1:104-143.

Freud, A. (1949), On certain difficulties in the preadolescent's relation to his parents. *The Writings of Anna Freud*, Vol. IV, 1968, IUP.

Freud, S. (1912), The dynamics of transference. *S.E.*, 12.

Freud, S. (1937), Analysis terminable and interminable. *S.E.*, 23.

Gill, M. M. (1979), The analysis of the transference. *J. Amer. Psychoanal. Assn.*, 27 (Suppl.) :263-288.

Kohrman, R. et al. (1971), Technique of child analysis: problems of countertransference. *Inter. J. Psycho-Anal.*, 52:487-497.

Kurosawa, Akira (1951), RASHOMON, a classic film.

Lipton, S.D. (1971), Freud's analysis of the Rat man considered as a technical paradigm. *Bull. Philad. Ass. Psychoanal.*, 21:179-183.

Lipton, S.D. (1977), The advantages of Freud's technique as shown in his analysis of the Rat Man, *Int. J. Psycho-Anal.*, 58:255-273.

Nagera, H. (1966), *Early Childhood Disturbances, The Infantile Neurosis And The Adulthood Disturbances: Problems of a Developmental Psychoanalytic Psychology*. New York: IUP. Monograph No. 2 of The Psychoanalytic Study of the Child.

National Committee for the Prevention of Child Abuse (1991), CHILD OF RAGE–A STORY OF CHILD ABUSE. An HBO documentary.

Racker, H. (1968), *Transference And Countertransference*. New York: IUP.

Solnit, A. (1987), It's never too late–new perspectives on child abuse. A paper presented at a conference in Chicago sponsored by the Juvenile Protective Association.

Weiss, S. (1964), Parameters in child analysis. *J. Amer. Psychoanal. Assn*, 12:587-599.

Weiss, S. et al. (1968), Technique of child analysis: problems of the opening phase. *J. Amer. Acad. Child Psychiat.*, 7:639-662.

Winnicott, D.W. (1958), *Collected Papers. Through Paediatrics to Psychoanalysis*. New York: Basic Books, Inc.

Countertransference Reactions in Death and Divorce: Comparison and Contrast

Benjamin Garber, MD

INTRODUCTION

The work with parents as an adjunct to the child's treatment has been a topic greatly neglected in the child psychiatric and psychoanalytic literature. Although the importance of working with parents has been recognized since the analysis of Little Hans (Freud 1905), there has not been any systematic exposition of how one deals with the parents of the child in treatment.

While it is generally assumed that some form of therapeutic intervention with parents will facilitate the child's therapy (Smirnoff, 1971; Glenn, 1978; Hoffman, 1984) the optimum method for doing so has remained elusive and idiosyncratic. Every therapist has a unique approach in dealing with parents. This evolves experientially and is influenced by each one's development as a parent and as a therapist of children. While such approaches may be inherently useful in individual circumstances they are not supported by a solid theoretical position nor by an empirical clinical data base.

Just as every therapeutic encounter is uniquely different, the parental interplay in and around the child's treatment is unique and diverse. Each parent brings a history, psychopathology, hopes and aspirations for the child to bear on the therapeutic process. Because of such diversity, it may well be that a variety of therapeutic models need to be developed to conceptualize the work with parents. At this stage in our history there are no viable theoretical models to help organize our thinking in this area. There is no consensus on the optimum method of dealing with parents in and around the treatment of the child. While there may be many reasons for such absences, I would like to suggest that our countertransference reactions to parents is one of the primary reasons that such efforts have lagged behind. Consequently we may consider the possibility that our countertransference reactions to the parents have become a significant interference in conceptualizing therapeutic strategies.

Although countertransference always comes from the therapist, a countertransference response is triggered by the psychopathology of the patient or some other element of the treatment situation. Therefore countertransference is usually the result of a fit between the needs of the therapist and the needs of the patient.

In the broad sense countertransference is defined as the response to a patient's transference with the analyst's own transference (Bernstein and Glenn 1988). While in recent times countertransference has been recognized as a potentially useful therapeutic tool, it is nevertheless a significant deviation from the optimal neutral therapeutic stance (Marcus 1980).

At various times all possible behavior and reactions to the patient on the part of the analyst have been labeled as countertransference. Kohrman et al. (1971) conceptualized all of the counter-behavior of the analyst in the generic sense as counterreactions. He spoke of a universal countertransference as a total response of the child analyst to the patient, the parents and the therapeutic situation. Countertransference proper was defined as the spontaneously occurring unconscious reaction of the analyst to the patient's transference which is quite specific and originates in the unresolved conflicts which complement those of the patient.

The therapeutic process with the child is set-up in a way that is bound to elicit countertransference responses to the parents. The child therapist sees the patient's parents as well as the patient. The therapist is in the middle of a family situation and he develops relationships with all of the family members.

The practical reality is that parents usually must be kept favorably disposed to a child's treatment if it is to continue and to progress. This may raise a troublesome conflict for a therapist who either competes with the parents or over-identifies with the child who may have been poorly parented. Transference reactions to the parents and identification with the child are extremely likely throughout the therapeutic process. For the therapist looks at the world from the child's point of view and tries to understand the patient's attitudes toward parents and other people. The therapist identifies with the patient empathically evoking memories of parental relationships from childhood (Olden 1953).

While as therapists we have many functions vis-à-vis the parents, our purpose is to understand the child, the parents' dreams for the child, and to be able to interpret the child to the parents. If we can accomplish these goals then there is the assumption that our goals for the treatment will more or less parallel the goals of the parents.

One of the best predictors of a successful treatment is parental support which translates as the parent's general understanding of the treatment process. For the parents to assist the child in continuing in treatment they must have a working alliance with the therapist. The alliance with the parents is set in motion during the diagnostic process and will give support for whatever treatment modality may be recommended. While such an alliance is hoped for, it is my contention that often our countertransference reactions become its greatest interference.

Every clinical situation has its own set of transference patterns and countertransference responses. The nature of these responses is in large part determined by the personalities, histories and psychopathology of the differing individuals. In this instance the focus will be on some of the transference interactions in situations of divorce and the death of a parent. These are two unique clinical situations which while similar in some respects, elicit a range of counter-reactions to the parents which are quite different from each other. I am hopeful that an attempt to spell out the specifics in particular clinical situations will shed some light on the work with parents and assist us in neutralizing the intensity of countertransference reactions.

COUNTERTRANSFERENCE IN DEATH AND DIVORCE

The child whose parent has died and the child whose parents have been divorced are viewed by society and therapists as unique victims of circumstance. In one instance by fate and in the other by seemingly unconcerned parents, the child has been dealt a cruel blow over which he or she has limited control. Consequently such children are looked at as victims who are in need of care, attention and support. Such youngsters will elicit our deepest concern and sympathy as we tend to overprotect them and make special allowances for them.

The concern for the child in death and divorce may have similar origins but reactions to the parents in each instance begin to diverge. It is these divergences that become the focus of intense countertransference reactions.

In parent loss, when a child is brought for an evaluation, the most frequent overt reason for referral is a need by the surviving parent to determine if the child is intact and if the parent is dealing reasonably well with the crisis. These parents want affirmation as to whether they are doing an adequate job of parenting under adverse circumstances. They see their situation as one of underlying emotional health but that fate has been less than kind to them. They approach the therapist from a position of emotional stability. Apart from an initial affirmation and advice there is scant motivation for long term intervention. The repetitive assertion is that prior to the loss, life was perfect, the lost parent was exceptional and psychopathology was non-existent. It is only since the death that some emotional problems may have appeared. In parent loss situations it is impossible to reconstruct a history of pre-loss psychopathology.

In the past it was fashionable to suggest that almost every child who experienced the loss of a parent needs to be in treatment (Furman 1974). In recent years this position has shifted to the point where we respect the surviving parent's and the bereaved child's innate adaptive capabilities. In part this clinical decision is based on the aforementioned history and in part it is based on the recognition that at the beginning of bereavement, the family's priorities do not include therapy. Perhaps at some later point a re-evaluation would be useful and then perhaps the issue of treatment will be reconsidered. I may add that such an approach with the Barr-Harris population has been inherently useful and therapeutically practical (Altschul 1988).

In divorce the initial presentation is different. The referral is usually the result of the child being in conflict with the environment. There has been a lengthy pre-divorce history of conflict and strife which has come to a head. Each parent recounts in detail the numerous flaws and deficits of the other parent. There is a marked emphasis on psychopathology and conflict. Consequently they enter the diagnostic process from a position of defectiveness. Their expectation is that the therapist should correct this flawed product from a flawed marriage. Their position is pathology-oriented and their expectations are unrealistic. There is an awareness by the therapist that this is only the beginning of a long and painful process of conflict and strife. The conflicts continue after the divorce with the potential entry of new partners. There may be an initial therapeutic expectation of a long term process with many disruptions.

As a result there is a tendency to see the bereaved parent as more intact and as someone who may need temporary assistance to cope with a crisis. In divorce there may be an immediate assumption of psychopathology which may or may not be valid. There is an immediate assumption of a parental lack of cooperation which may be equally invalid. The work of Cohen, Cohler and Weissman (1984) has demonstrated that there are situations where parents may be at odds with each other about most matters but that a parenting alliance may exist where the needs of the child are considered. Nevertheless the dye is cast from the initial contact and the diagnostic process may suffer from countertransference intrusions.

In the beginning in parent loss, it is easy to marshal our empathic capacities and to respond appropriately and therapeutically to the trauma. We may experience a profound sadness when listening to the details of the loss. Within therapeutic limits, we may grieve with the surviving parent and bereaved child. Such responses, if maintained within certain bounds, are appropriate and therapeutic. These responses let the surviving parent know that we feel for them, that we comprehend their pain and that we are therapeutically attuned to their distress. These responses let them know that while we can feel what they feel, we can also stand back and frame the situation in its proper clinical context. Whatever the outcome, in the beginning we are moved by their distress.

In divorce, the diagnostic response may be quite different. We listen to each parent's distress, unhappiness, disappointment and pain. We recognize the conflicts and we try to make sense of what went wrong and how it may have affected the child. However after listening to the repetitive nature of the complaints, we may experience a subtle irritation and a growing annoyance with these two adults who are enmeshed in an all consuming struggle. In their regressed state, they have forgotten the child. We have to suppress the wish to moralize, to criticize and to highlight destructive tendencies. In order to avoid such counter-reactions we are likely to retreat to an overly intellectualized clinical stance. Consequently our empathic capacities are compromised from the beginning.

As clinicians we experience a variety and range of counter-transference reactions. The ones that are most likely to be noticed are those involving anger, hate or fear because they are the most likely to cause anxiety in the therapist. In order not to experience and not to deal with such affect we find means to avoid the parents of our child patients.

According to Childress (1988) a misrepresentation of the classic analytic model can be used to distance ourselves from parents who make us anxious. It is less easy to see treatment itself as an intrusion into the family and our own aloofness, unavailability, criticism, exasperation and even discourtesy as a problem.

Since divorced parents are the most eager to maintain contact with the therapist they are also the most likely to be avoided. Divorced parents call often to complain about the ex-spouse, his or her misdeeds, destructiveness or manipulations. These are complaints that the therapist has heard many times. Since there is no constructive response to such a litany then there is no choice but to listen one more time to the hatreds, disappointments and resentments that have destroyed the marriage.

Since there are no culturally prescribed laws or rituals how one should deal with the various complications that arise around the daily living situation in divorce the parent may call because of confusion and a lack of knowledge. Yet we assume that they are usually calling to complain about the ex-spouse or the child. Consequently there is a tendency to limit and minimize contacts in a situation where just the opposite may be necessary.

In divorce it is easy to rationalize such avoidances because we assume that the parents, especially the non-custodial ones, are not that interested nor concerned about the child. There may evolve a subtle pact between custodial parent and therapist whereby the other parent is excluded from all contacts and meaningful communication. Such avoidances may be based on a phantasy that the therapist will become a better parent to the child than the non-custodial disinterested partner. While the custodial parent may indeed collude in such acting-out it is difficult for us to empathize with the sense of loss and shame that is experienced by the loser in custody wars.

In situations where a parent has died the initial contacts with the therapist by the surviving parent may be frequent as there are questions about the proper time to initiate certain activities. As the therapy progresses, contacts with the therapist diminish as the parent begins to "get on with life." In fact the parent tends to avoid the therapist, for such encounters serve as viable reminders of a loss which may elicit a profound emotional response.

We comply with such avoidances and minimize communication with the surviving parent but for different reasons. We assume that the parent has followed our instructions and suggestions faithfully so that there is no need to emphasize and repeat the obvious. Parents will tell us that they have heard it all before and that they know what to do so that further meetings are not necessary. While parents' avoidance motives are not to be reminded of the loss, the therapist's avoidance may have to do with an idealization of the surviving parent. Just the way the parent idealizes the one that died, we idealize the survivors because of their seeming ability to negotiate one of life's greatest traumas.

The informational framework consists of the therapist knowing what is going on with the parent and/or parents in death and in divorce. Gathering this information will stimulate significant countertransference reactions.

When a child's parent dies there is an awareness of when and how it happened. The events of the death and the resulting family shifts are generally known and recognized. The surviving parent's adaptation to the loss is noted, and while the community may not necessarily agree on the proper length of a viable mourning process it is generally agreed that after a certain amount of time life has to go on. Mourning rituals are religiously and culturally prescribed and are carried out within a defined time frame. Anniversaries are noted and reacted to as there is a general awareness of the basic elements of a mourning process.

In divorce the process and its significant landmarks remain fuzzy. The community at large may not know just when the separation occurred. Indirectly, it may be found out when a parent has moved out or when the parent returned to the household. The finality of the divorce is always a moot point and left to much speculation and conjecture. The appearance of a replacement for the absent parent is also not clear so that much of what really transpires in the household of divorce is left to speculation and phantasy. This speculative and uncertain stance is buttressed by each parent's accusation of the other for withholding information about activities, timetables and finances. Each parent will accuse the other of withholding significant data and each parent may suggest the therapist's stupidity at being duped by the other. Not only is significant and important information withheld about each other, but also about the child. The patient may be suddenly shifted from one household to another, from one school to another, and not infrequently from one therapist to another. The therapeutic process with such a youngster is full of surprises.

While this lack of information and frequent surprises may stimulate anger in the therapist there are also phantasies about the nature of the sexual acting-out of each partner. These phantasies may be fueled and supported by rival accusations and innuendoes.

Because of a lack of information and because of a constant parental conscious and unconscious withholding, the therapist functions in an informational vacuum. Consequently there may be surprises as to what is really going on and as to who does what to whom and when. The therapist is kept off balance about the latest move and maneuver by either parent. Such lack of information will contribute to the therapist's anger at both parents and will lend a precariousness to the treatment. It would seem that the precariousness of the whole undertaking is an ever present accompaniment of one's work with the child of divorce.

The child whose parent has died is frequently the recipient of much support from the immediate and extended families as well as the community at large. There is much sympathy and empathy for the child and the surviving parent. Family members may assist with short term caretaking, religion offers comforting rituals, teachers may make special allowances and community resources are made available to the surviving parent. In the short run and sometimes for the duration, the surviving parent is not alone. Such resources are essential for adaptation and may indeed have a significant impact on outcome and psychopathology (Garber 1984).

A completely opposite situation evolves in divorce as from the beginning the immediate and extended families have divided into warring camps. The sides have been chosen based on blood ties and assignation of blame. Since the parents are held to blame for the imposed disruption, there is little empathy, support or assistance from the community. The mutual hatred and bitterness contributes to a discomfort which is often expressed in avoidance. Consequently the divorcing parents remain more or less isolated and have to marshal their own resources. The surrounding network may not only be unresponsive but may accuse and condemn the parents for their selfishness and lack of concern for the child. There may evolve a situation in which each parent stakes out a territory in the community and creates a shell of protectiveness in order to avoid the accusations and rumors. Such avoidances are laced with a protective hostility and cynicism which may be transmitted to the child. It is not uncommon for the child of divorce to present in treatment as cynical, suspicious and mistrustful, a necessary protection not only from the parental crossfire, but also from the community at large.

Because of the constant anger, fear of retaliation or the danger of being accused of taking sides, we as therapists also avoid the divorcing parents. Because of an exaggerated neutrality we keep our distance, because of studied impartiality we communicate little and in this way contribute to the divorcing parents isolation. We also condemn and accuse, not necessarily in ways that are overtly destructive, but in a distancing from the conflict which can be interpreted as rejection. In a sense we are members of the community which is at odds with the divorcing parents and the child in their midst.

In working with a child who has experienced the loss of a parent, the therapeutic task is relatively straightforward. It is to assist the child in experiencing some type of mourning process that is in keeping with his or her developmental capabilities (Garber 1981). The treatment goals can be presented with certainty and directness to the surviving parent. Whether the child and/or surviving parent choose to accept these goals is another matter. Nevertheless as therapists we have a clear cut idea as to what needs to be done and these expectations can be spelled out to parent and child. We also possess a vast body of clinical data and a theoretical framework to organize this data. We are on solid ground in prescribing a treatment regimen based on an appreciation of what constitutes a reasonable and appropriate mourning process. While much of our work with children is vague and uncertain, there is a consensus that mourning is essential for development to proceed. Psychoanalytic work with children (Furman 1974) and adults (Fleming and Altschul 1968) support such assumptions. Although there are numerous models of mourning from differing frames of reference there is little argument that mourning is essential for emotional well being, adaptation and stability.

In divorce the therapeutic goals become more vague and uncertain. It is important for the child to come to terms with the divorce, however, operationally it is not clear just what that means or what it may involve. In divorce just as in loss by death, the child is expected to mourn something but the elements of that mysterious something are not clear. The child does not necessarily mourn the absent parent, but needs to mourn the pre-divorce intact family constellation and to relinquish the image and the phantasy of the intact family which will never be there again.

The child is also expected to deal with the various affects in regard to the divorce, the sadness, shame, the guilt and most importantly the anger. However for the therapist, the therapeutic task becomes rather vague because instead of dealing with internally constituted issues with which we are cognizant and comfortable, we are put in the unfamiliar position of mediators. Because of the ongoing strife, we are forced out of our traditional role and instead we have to mediate disputes. These disputes may involve the child and each parent, the parents themselves or the child and the environment. Our internally focused orientation is swept aside and we are forced into unfamiliar externally oriented territory. In such instances we may become unsure, vague, helpless and probably quite anxious. Our expertise is demeaned as we are confronted with warring parties demanding a solution to an insoluble problem. Our narcissism is injured as once again there is a tendency to withdraw and contribute to the parental aloneness.

Because of being cast in an untraditional and unfamiliar role, we tend to become angry at the involved parties or to withdraw and to rationalize that we are confronted with an unworkable situation.

In the treatment of the bereaved child, we often tend to slip out of our neutral therapeutic stance and find ourselves becoming a real person to the child. This may manifest itself clinically when the child asks innocent questions about the therapist's outside life. In order not to deprive the traumatized youngster, we answer. The child may want the therapist to replace the dead parent while we see a viable possibility of rescuing the child. We phantasize about replacing the lost parent only we will do a more competent job of parenting. We may react to such wishes by becoming and acting overly moral with the surviving parent and child or by becoming overly supportive and controlling of the surviving parent. As a result there may be a tendency to become overly involved with the parent or to realize that involvement and to withdraw. In either instance it is a function of the wish to replace the absent parent. Such behavior will certainly dovetail with the child's need to seek a replacement and of the parent's need to find a new partner, especially if the therapist is the same sex as the parent that died.

In divorce the issues are similar but also different only in the sense that we wish to rescue the child from both of these flawed individuals. In so doing, we may turn the child against the parents by emphasizing their deficits, or by emphasizing that if it were up to us we would do it differently and certainly better. Such behavior may dovetail with child's and parent's initial expectations and idealizations. In either instance the motivation is to rescue the child and to replace the parents as well as to offer the child a perfect nonjudgmental parent and friend: perhaps something that we have always longed for ourselves.

One of the common countertransference problems that emerges in the treatment of parent loss is the making of special allowances which foster a moving away from and distortion of the treatment contract. The basic interaction in any therapeutic process vacillates around the to and fro of the treatment contract which is spelled out in the beginning. The verbal agreement about the mutual responsibilities of patient and therapist constitute the essence of the practical framework around which the therapy is organized.

When working with a parent loss case, there is a greater tendency to overlook the elements of the original contract. Such issues as missed appointments, charging for missed appointments or not adhering to the agreed upon frequency are just a few of the day to day transactions that tend to be overlooked. Such oversights are usually rationalized under the general category of a realistic appreciation of the hardships encountered by a parent whose life has been disrupted by the loss. They may also be looked at as expressions of sympathy for a parent who has experienced an overwhelming trauma.

While such oversights may be appreciated in the short run they have a debilitating effect on the solidification and continuity of the process. It is not uncommon for the treatment to begin to flounder because of the many disruptions. The only viable process is one of half-hearted fits and stops which interfere with progress. The therapist may then be confronted by an angry parent who demands a progress report and who not infrequently terminates the treatment.

In divorce there are also significant deviations from the original contract, however, these are usually beyond the control of the therapist. Nevertheless, they elicit anger at the divorcing parents which is then displaced to the child.

In the work with the child of divorce, appointments are missed, conferences are avoided and bills are not paid as there is an unconscious attempt by the non-custodial parent to disrupt the treatment while the custodial parent may not have the energy to overcome such obstacles. There seem to be legitimate reasons for the disruptions and they invariably have their roots in one parent's anger towards the other. Such disruptions are a blow to the therapist's self-esteem who is engaged in a therapeutic push and pull with a resistant passive-aggressive child.

Since the parents cannot be engaged except in a dialogue in which they express only anger at each other then the therapist is put in a position of helplessness and rage. Being angry at each parent the therapist is then in a position of identification with the helpless child. While experiencing a taste and feel of what the child has to contend with the therapist is reduced to a helpless victim who can vent frustration only at the child who happens to be there.

For the child of divorcing parents every interaction is permeated with loyalty conflicts. Every decision within the disintegrating family involves loyalty considerations. The child's loyalty conflicts are a major contributory element to the psychopathology for they tend to destroy the child's relationship to both parents (Garber 1984).

The therapist may also experience loyalty conflicts with allegiance shifting from one parent to the other. Initially the therapist may experience greater empathy and compassion for the parent of the same sex, however that may shift as the treatment progresses. At a later time the therapist may feel more loyal to the parent who is more supportive of the treatment and may then focus on the deficits of the less supportive one. Loyalty and identification are closely related so that the therapist may alternately identify with each parent's position.

Such shifting identifications may become unsettling so that ultimately the therapist may move to a position of greater detachment and distance in order to preserve even-handedness. Such shifts by the therapist may confuse the child in his or her loyalty struggles, for the therapist is expected to remain neutral. These shifts may be equally confusing to the parents as each one will attempt to ally with the therapist against the other. Frantic attempts by each parent to enlist the therapist's loyalty may lead to a greater detachment and withdrawal. Parents may be quick to seize on such inconsistencies and confront the therapist in a most uncomfortable manner.

In parent loss the conflict centers around preserving loyalty to the parent that died. How quickly should the surviving parent date and remarry involves loyalty considerations toward the one that died. If we feel that the surviving parent is planning to date and to remarry prematurely there may be a tendency to lecture and to moralize about the importance of remembering. We may labor excessively in the service of keeping the memory of the dead parent alive. There may be anger at the surviving parent which may be presented as the wish to avoid mourning. We may insist on memorialization and remembering in a way that may not be reasonable and appropriate. For while remembering the dead parent is important it should be in a way that is spontaneous and ego-syntonic to parent and child.

It has long been debated whether one can treat a patient competently for whom one feels strong emotion such as love, hate, fear or anger. These countertransference reactions give us some explanation of why the therapeutic work in divorce is so difficult and demanding. Our empathic capacities for the grieving parent usually remain intact. It is not difficult to empathize with grieving parents in their sadness and sense of loss. It is equally easy to be empathic with the parents' lament about the unfairness of it all. Such feelings are part and parcel of the human condition. We are most likely to lose our empathic stance when the parent denies the importance of the loss or wishes to short circuit the mourning process by quickly finding a replacement and by withdrawing the child from treatment (Garber 1989). Such parental denials are most likely to elicit our wrath and condemnation. Such a reaction is partly based on some type of culturally and emotionally predetermined timetable about the proper length of mourning and a respectable time to wait before remarrying. Such anger at the surviving parent may give us license to make dire predictions about the child's future since the mourning work was not completed.

Once again our competitiveness with the parent may carry the day for we are implying that if this were our child we would do it differently and certainly better. We would persist in the push and pull of the treatment process until the child is forced to mourn in compliance with an adultomorphic model of mourning.

There is an assumption that a hasty replacement for the dead parent is doomed to failure. We are unable to consider the possibility that if the child and parent are unable or even unwilling to deal with the loss now they will be able to go back and do so at some later time in their development. Consequently some terminations will be abrupt and filled with mutual recrimination and withdrawal. We tend to lose sight of the fact that an unfavorable termination may preclude the option and shut the door to the possibility that will allow the parent and child to come back and mourn at a later time. Once again in our competitiveness with parent there may be a preconscious wish for the child to fail just so we can point to our predictions with a sense of self-righteousness and self-justification.

Therapists invariably feel sad about terminations, a sign of their transferences. In parent loss situations this feeling may be compounded since it is also a response to the patient's sadness which may be great as they are re-experiencing the original trauma. To avoid such powerful affects it is not surprising that in the treatment of parent loss the termination phase may become abbreviated. This may be one instance in which the therapist identifies with the surviving parent and wishes to avoid experiencing the powerful feelings of sadness about the loss.

In divorce our ability to empathize is compromised from the beginning. It is primarily the anger at the destructive uncaring self-centered and interfering parents that hampers our empathic capacities. We dread meetings with each or both parents as much time will be spent listening to each one's bitter complaints about the other. We bemoan the fact that concerns for the child's well being are shunted aside in the service of personal vendettas and so we are relieved when such encounters end.

Since the child's treatment is equally rocky because of parental lack of support and because we displace our anger from the unavailable parents to an angry, sullen passive-aggressive child, then it may not be surprising that we experience a sense of relief when the treatment finally ends. The parents may experience similar feelings as they wish to get away from this distant, withdrawn aloof and critical therapist who is equally flawed. Then they proceed to the next easily idealized therapist. This one will fix their flawed product. Unfortunately each experience only highlights and emphasizes the defectiveness of parent and child as neither could be properly fixed.

Having been devalued by angry parents who are disappointed at our not having fixed their flawed product and devalued by the cynical withdrawn child who would rather do other things, we experience a re-establishment of self-esteem when we dismiss such a family as untreatable. Unplanned and abrupt terminations for which absent finances are the common rationalization are frequent in the treatment of children of divorce. Even the last few sessions so essential for a sense of closure are often avoided by both parties with a sense of mutual relief. Unfortunately the parents may continue the same quest with another therapist while we proceed to treat the next child of divorce knowing full well that reality circumstances and our countertransferences will contribute to a most difficult treatment encounter.

CONCLUSION

In the subjective world of individual insight oriented psychotherapy it is almost impossible to make comparisons and to draw conclusions from a comparison between the therapeutic approaches with two different types of problems such as the impact of divorce and the death of a parent on the child.

However, there are some clues in the psychiatric literature which may assist in comparing the two populations. Rutter (1971) found that the loss of a parent by separation or divorce was more traumatic and longer lasting than loss by death. In a comparison of delinquency studies (Rutter 1971) it was found that the rates of delinquency were nearly double for boys whose parents had divorced or separated as compared with no parental loss but only slightly elevated when the boys had lost a parent by death. In a study of adolescent girls self-esteem was higher in girls who lost a parent by death than those who lost a parent by separation or divorce (Heathrighton, 1972).

While there are many factors that would explain such differences we would have to assume that there is something about our countertransference responses to the parents in each instance that may impact on the treatment outcome in death and in divorce.

It is clear from both the controlled studies and uncontrolled reports that parental influences are closely related to the degree and nature of change in many children (Simmons 1981). So that if in our contact with the parents we are unable to assess, set aside or use our countertransference reactions constructively then it is bound to have a negative impact on the outcome of the work with the child.

Children of divorce seem to be adversely affected by continuous turbulent relationships between the parents and parents' forbidding the child contact with the absent parent. By the same token these children are also affected adversely by a turbulent relationship between the therapist and the parents. For such replays in the treatment situation may be the rule rather than the exception.

There is little doubt that the child will gain if the therapist has a good working relationship with the parents. Whether the parents are in treatment or whether there is a good informational alliance both are essential for the parents' ability to sustain the therapy in the face of the child's resistance.

Just the way it is essential for the child's development and well-being to maintain contact with both parents in divorce and to remember the parent that died, in a parallel fashion it is essential for the therapist to maintain ongoing contact with the parent in order that the treatment process may unfold and develop. For ultimately it is for the benefit of the child so that an attempt to set aside our countertransference reactions may indeed be for the best interest of the child.

REFERENCES

Altschul, S. (1988) *Childhood Bereavement and its Aftermath.* International Universities Press: Madison, CT.

Bernstein, I, and J. Glen (1988) The child and adolescent analyst's emotional reactions to his patients and their parents. *International Review of Psychoanalysis.* 15:225-241.

Childress, B. (1988) Working with parents and the diagnostic process. *ACP Newsletter.* 3:11-13.

Cohen, R., Cohler, B. and S. Weissman (1984) *Parenthood A Psychodynamic Perspective.* The Guilford Press: New York.

Fleming, J. and S. Altschul (1963) Activation of mourning and growth. *International Journal of Psychoanalysis.* 44:419-431.

Freud, S. (1905) Analysis of a phobia in a five year old boy. *Standard Edition.* 10:3-149. Hogarth Press: London. 1953.

Furman, E. (1974) *A Child's Parent Dies: Studies in Childhood Bereavement.* Yale University Press: New Haven, CT.

Garber, B. (1981) Mourning in Children: Toward a theoretical synthesis. *The Annual of Psychoanalysis.* 9:9-19. International Universities Press: New York.

Garber, B. (1984) Parenting responses in divorce and bereavement of a spouse. In (Eds) Cohen, R., Cohler, B. and S. Weissman. *Parenthood: A Psychodynamic Perspective.* Guilford Press: New York.

Garber, B. (1988) Some common transference countertransference issues in the treatment of parent loss. In [Ed] Altschul, S., *Childhood Bereavement and its Aftermath.* International Universities Press: New York, pp. 137-152.

Garber, B. (1989) The child's mourning: Can it be learned from the parent. In [Eds] Field, K., Cohler, B., and G. Wool, *Learning and Education: Psychoanalytic Perspectives.* IUP: Madison, CT. pp 355-377.

Glenn, J. (1978) *Child Analysis and Therapy.* Jason Aronson: New York.

Hetherington, E.M. (1972) Effects of father absence on personality development in adolescent daughters. *Developmental Psychology.* 7:213-226.

Hoffman, M. (1984) The parent's experience with the child's therapist. In [Eds] Cohen, R., Cohler, B., and S. Weissman. *Parenthood a Psychodynamic Perspective.* Guilford Press: New York. pp. 164-172.

Kohrman, R. et al. (1971) Techniques of child analysis. Problems of countertransference. *International Journal of Psychoanalysis.* 52:487-497.

Marcus, I. (1980) Countertransference and the psychoanalytic process in children and adolescents. *The Psychoanalytic Study of the Child.* Vol. 35. Yale University Press: New Haven, CT.

Olden, C. (1953) On adult empathy with children. *The Psychoanalytic Study of the Child.* Vol. 8. International Universities Press: New York.

Rutter, M. (1971) Parent child separation: Psychological effects on the children. *Journal Child Psychology and Psychiatry.* 12:233-260.

Simmons, I. (and others) (1981) Parent treatability: What is it? *Journal American Academy of Child Psychiatry.* 20:4. 785-788.

Smirnoff, V. (1971) *The Scope of Child Analysis.* International Universities Press: New York.

Countertransference Problems in Dealing with Severely Disturbed Parents: Their Potential Value for Understanding the Patient

M. Barrie Richmond, MD

INTRODUCTION

This paper was initially stimulated by Jacqui Sanders' concern about our need for a deeper understanding of the problematic parental alliances that regularly recur in dealing diagnostically and therapeutically with very troubled children and adolescents. This neglected subject interests me a great deal, in part because it allows a certain freedom of thought in investigating the organizing role of the distinctive countertransferences and counterresistances evoked by this patient group (as compared with less seriously disturbed patients with neurotic and narcissistic character psychopathology).

From the three illustrative composite clinical cases that follow, I will discuss the use of the analyst's countertransference as an organizer to formulate the diagnostic and therapeutic process in dealing with severely disturbed (psychotic) patients and their families. Three prominent psychodynamic themes will be stressed: the influence of dependency conflicts; competitive parental envy; and the process of identification with the aggressor. These themes may operate either separately or in combination with each other to influence the therapeutic process as the psychoanalyst tries to deal effectively with these children and their parents.

The use of the word "patient" in the title of this paper requires clarification. The word patient includes children, adolescents and also adults in their late 20's (whom I think of developmentally as late adolescents) because they are still overly-dependent on their parents emotionally and financially. The analyst is, in a parallel process way, analogously dependent on the parents' cooperation and support.

My clinical and theoretical ideas–especially the conceptual language employed–derive from varied sources, including my personal analysis, child and adolescent psychoanalytic training, and the insights and recommendations of several colleagues who have facilitated my understanding of the problems that arise in dealing with severely disturbed patients and their parents. Part of my purpose in presenting this paper is to assert my conviction that these patients and parents cause difficult countertransferences for all psychoanalysts.

PARALLEL PROCESS AND COUNTERIDENTIFICATION

The poet, John Keats, in elaborating his conception of "negative capability," wrote that the man of poetic imagination was characterized by his openness to new formative experiences–experiences essential to pursuing truth. I have been interested in the use of counteridentification as a means of dealing with the problems associated with following the diagnostic and therapeutic process with severely disturbed patients. Beginning with my first adult control case as a psychoanalytic candidate, I became convinced of the value of utilizing the parallel process perspective to clarify the patient's otherwise ununderstandable feeling state. My first control supervisor, at the conclusion of an unusually difficult series of hours, pointed out that my patient was feeling as helpless and as hopeless as I appeared to be feeling.

As I began to consider the parallel process perspective in relation to the countertransference counteridentifications evoked in me by parents of very disturbed children and adolescents, I gradually came to the realization that the blocked affects and perceptual distortions of these severely disturbed patients resisted standard attempts to understand the therapeutic process; however, by shifting my attention to clarifying the evoked countertransference, I found that the patient's experience became more intelligible. This perspective provided a crucial opportunity to understand the dysphoric feelings and upsetting thoughts that I would have preferred to resist about the child, his parents and myself–especially when irrational or psychotic (Bion) anxieties were being mobilized.

BION'S CONCEPTUAL LANGUAGE

Bion's conceptual language and views about the thought processes of very disturbed patients can be useful in clarifying the psychoanalyst's countertransference. Bion's ideas about the psychotic personality form an essential link–to use his language–for understanding how catastrophic anxiety, reversal of perspective and other psychotic fears are experienced and mobilized in the patient, parents and the psychoanalyst in response to these psychotic mechanisms and processes. He uses the term psychotic personality to refer to a distinct form of mental functioning that becomes evident in the (manifest) clinical content involving the patient's language and behaviour as well as in the psychoanalyst's induced response [e.g., as part of the process of projective identification]. According to Bion, the psychotic personality form of functioning co-exists with the non-psychotic personality mode of thinking and behavior. In considering therapeutic work with severely disturbed patients, the key issue for Bion in evaluating patients is: Which mode of functioning predominates? In severely disturbed children, adolescents and their parents the psychotic personality mode predominates and is apparent in the patient's or parent's psychological disorganization and instability [of the thought processes] (Grinberg et al., p. 27, 1977).

Bion also contends that the psychotic processes which he describes as a form of mental functioning [rather than a diagnostic entity] are ubiquitous. Accordingly, the psychoanalyst must deal with the activation of his own repressed psychotic processes when dealing with these severely disturbed children, adolescents and their parents.

THE USE OF COUNTERTRANSFERENCE
WITH SEVERELY DISTURBED PATIENTS

Due to the severity of their disturbance, the child and adolescent patients and parents that I am discussing are unable to form helpful therapeutic and parental alliances. Countertransference tensions that are specifically related to the patient's or parent's psychopathology invariably arise with these patients. The psychoanalyst is frequently frustrated in his attempts at analysis or intensive insight-oriented psychoanalytic psychotherapy. When we listen to a child, adolescent, or his parent (in the absence of this type of countertransference tension—with its implicit pressure to act) we are usually able to maintain our interest in answering the structural theory question, what's the patient's intrapsychic conflict? Structural theory focuses on unconscious conflict and resolution of the patient's compromise formations. As we carefully observe the patients we treat from the structural theory perspective, we try to understand the meaning of the child's or adolescent's associations and their relationship to the analytic or therapeutic situation. Our answer to the question posed requires an assessment of the context of the analytic situation, i.e., the state of the transference; the genetic-dynamic meaning behind the content expressed, etc.

At a recent meeting of the American Psychoanalytic Association (1985), Jacob Arlow pointed out some of the important assumptions and implications behind the structural theory's approach for organizing clinical experiences. The psychoanalyst, as a first step, organizes a narrative summary of the patient's clinical content around basic neurotic psychoanalytic themes, e.g., separation; competitiveness, submission, etc. However, as I have stated earlier, a problem arises when we are dealing with psychotic processes (e.g., deeply envious early oral greed conflicts) rather than neurotic processes (e.g., post-oedipal conflictual competitive tensions) that can usually be understood and analyzed by the experienced clinician who follows structural theory. When the child's or adolescent's clinical content lacks affective meaning (Modell, 1990), the psychoanalyst cannot respond in an effective therapeutic manner.

The problems associated in dealing with severely disturbed patients and their parents are in large part due to the fact that frequently the psychoanalyst is not provided with useful clinical material such as dreams, play, associations or a narrative context as seen in well-differentiated neurotic characters. As a result, he is unable to formulate and interpret the therapeutic process; remarkably, he is rendered incapable of associating productively to the severely disturbed patient's play, dream, or verbal and non-verbal clinical material. Since the patient's clinical content is repressed, suppressed, or disavowed, it can only become available through enactments, symbolic actions, or other forms of unconscious acting out. Due to the boredom countertransference (Bernstein, 1990) evoked by the emptiness and lack of [thematic] meaning in the patient's communications, the psychoanalyst cannot formulate the patient's psychopathology unless he recognizes the crucial value of his countertransference tension as a signal function for providing the missing links necessary to clarify the genetic-dynamic background.

Clinical Case Illustrations

To introduce the clinical part of this paper, I want to make a brief comment about how I "position" myself in diagnostic and therapeutic work with severely disturbed children and adolescents. I am initially interested in observing the parental alliance and its expectable vicissisitudes. Accordingly, I evaluate from the first moment [e.g., the first phone call] that a child or adolescent is referred to me the impact on my psychological (emotional) equilibrium of the transactions that ensue while obtaining the patient's present history, developmental and family background. I anticipate that I will experience dysphoric feeling states of varying intensity evoked by the parents or the patient. These disturbances in my intrapsychic balance are indicated by so-called signal affects, e.g., anxiety, boredom, rage. In trying to observe how my psychological equilibrium is disrupted affectively by the patient or his parents, I find that these dysphoric feelings usually occur as a spontaneous reaction which is not necessarily linked directly to the [manifest] clinical content.

With both neurotic and more severely disturbed children and adolescents, I try to understand their feelings from the viewpoint of their antecedent genetic and current dynamic intrapsychic conflicts (Abrams, S. 1978). However, with the more severely disturbed children and adolescents, I find that the patient's clinical content doesn't provide meaningful information about his/her inner experiences and thus I am unable to formulate the therapeutic process or make a complete transference diagnosis. In contrast, I find that with non-psychotic children, adolescents, and young adults standard interviewing technique is usually sufficient for eliciting interpretable, affectively meaningful clinical material (i.e., without countertransference analysis).

As an attempt to counter the omnipresent danger of imposing my adult view of reality on the child's experience and construction of reality (Modell, 1991b), I use the elicited countertransference experience as an organizer to formulate the diagnostic/therapeutic process and clarify the diagnosis of the transference. With more severely disturbed children and adolescents, I anticipate experiencing a parallel process counteridentification. In assuming the parallel process perspective, which I link to the expectable countertransference counteridentification, I anticipate that I will experience some variation (perhaps in derivative form) of how the child has been made to feel helpless and dependent, enraged, terrified, etc.

The child's feeling of helpless dependence has two important sources: the complete biological dependency on parents for survival and the control and compliance-defiance conflictual themes that derive from the mother infant dyad. As much as I may wish to empathize with the child's actual inner experiences, I realize that this goal can, at best, only be approximated. My dependency conflicts and feelings of helplessness may resonate closely with the child's experience, however, the reality and intensity of these feelings for the child results in a qualitatively different experience. On the other hand, I would not minimize the discomfort and tribulations the psychoanalyst experiences in dealing with intense, [often incompletely analyzed] helpless/dependent countertransference affects which are evoked by the child's or parent's unconscious projective identification. When these countertransference counteridentifications are mobilized, I assume that they confirm the child's feeling of helpless dependence. There is a crucial distinction: my reaction, when processed correctly, eventually seems manageable; whereas the child continues to experience his helplessness not as an intrapsychic conflict but as a menacing reality which, because of its traumatic intensity, leaves him overwhelmed [due to structural de-differentiation].

I assume the parallel process perspective and believe that the mother-infant dyad is recreated in a parallel way between the parent and the psychoanalyst. The parent controls and makes the therapist dependent on him/her in several ways: e.g., by bringing the pre-school or older child to sessions on time; by reminding the older child about the sessions; or negatively: delaying payment; not paying; threatening the end of treatment; precipitously withdrawing the child from treatment; threatening to disrupt or actually disrupting the therapist's practice; etc.

Clinical Case Illustration #1

This clinical example illustrates the themes of dependency, competitive envy, and identification with the aggressor as well as the mechanisms of reversal of perspective and catastrophic anxiety as formulated by Bion but without the analyst understanding how these theoretical perspectives clarify the diagnostic and therapeutic process.

A divorced, overbearing mother of a reportedly [by the boy's school] very disturbed nine year old Caucasian Catholic boy called to consult with me about psychotherapy for her son. In the course of the initial diagnostic interview with her, I indicated that her son might require frequent, insight-oriented psychotherapy sessions. She told me that the amount of therapy was out of her control; it was a matter that her son's father would have to decide about since he was the one who was financially responsible for all of their son's [medical and psychiatric] expenses. She gratuitously volunteered that I should expect some difficulty in payment–she complained that she had just concluded a prolonged divorce that cost her thousands of dollars in legal fees. As my anxiety titre dramatically increased, she also related in exquisite detail the subsequent "war-zone" experiences she had endured with her manipulative and controlling ex-husband. She warned me that since he was independently wealthy he would use his money to control me in whatever way he wished. Spontaneously, she suggested several ways that he might disrupt my practice–e.g., by ordering depositions; demanding extended court hearings; requiring periodic written reports for him to evaluate my work; and insisting on open-ended personal interviews with me irrespective of considerations concerning confidentiality or the time constraints of my practise.

Afterwards, when I reviewed what had happened during this interview, I was eventually able to reconstruct how she had controlled what had happened: somehow she had rendered me passive as she described in detail how manipulative and bullying her son's father had been to her (and would be to me). Later that day she phoned to complain that I seemed preoccupied with her ex-husband and questioned whether I was the right person for her son. A second interview was arranged to help her evaluate whether I was the right person for her son. During this session I realized that I was unwilling to deal with the mother's and father's psychopathology. I was not unaware of how uncomfortable the boy's mother made me feel; however, I still could not escape the intense, recurring feeling that I wanted to avoid this case. Regrettably, I acted on my feeling by telling the mother that if I were to work with her son I would have to insist that both parents be counseled about him by someone else since I had concluded that it would be essential for his treatment that confidentiality be maintained and therefore I would not be able to have any communication with either parent.

As I had anticipated, the boy's mother could not accept this loss of control and I was terminated shortly after this (second) session. She responded to my bill by paying for the first session only; she refused to pay for the second session which she deemed worthless. I sighed a sigh of relief. (Nor did I decide to hire a lawyer about the remaining balance and wage war with her as I thought she had invited me to do.)

For some time I was relieved that I had avoided this potential nightmare, despite my qualms about the fate of the boy. About four months later a colleague told me about a recent referral of the same boy–actually I had suggested my colleague's name to the boy's mother. He told me that he had taken the position with the mother that he was eager to meet the boy's father and that he would work with their son only if the father was completely happy with him. My colleague further reported that there were no problems in dealing with the father; however, the boy's mother eventually destroyed the therapy.

Of course, almost everything I had thought and done was wrong. At no time did I think of the parents as patients in their own right who needed a therapeutic response. Also, I had missed the opportunity to learn about the boy's relationships with his parents by considering my countertransference from the parallel process viewpoint. What I needed most, it seems to me, were clinical theory guidelines that would provide direction for dealing with these parents and processing such clinical experiences systematically to further my understanding of their son.

As a result of such devastating clinical experiences, I eventually came upon the idea of processing the content of diagnostic and therapeutic interviews in two different ways. When I feel comfortable I follow the standard theory of technique: I listen; pay attention to the verbal content; play with the child; associate to the material; ask clarifying questions; interpret dreams, symptoms and parapraxes; reconstruct the patient's narrative: and then summarize the content to formulate the therapeutic process around transference and resistance themes. In sharp contrast, whenever I begin to feel uncomfortable because I am beginning to experience a dysphoric affect, I more-or-less stop trying to do the above; instead, I pay careful attention to my own affective response–anger, fear, boredom, etc. I assume that the patient is either repressing/suppressing a thought or feeling or has "infected" me with a "virulent" projective identification. The effect of the patient's projective identification is typically a persistent thought or feeling that I can't get rid of–like a bad flu! I try to differentiate whether I am experiencing psychotic or non-psychotic affects to assess the impact of the projective identification mechanism. Since I have a fairly reliable set of defences–at least most of the time–I am quite capable of fending off psychotic anxieties like the terrible feeling of being terrorized that this boy's mother was generating in me. [As you can see, I haven't told you about the boy directly . . . or perhaps I have conveyed more about him to you than I wanted to know.]

In general, I believe that each psychoanalyst who treats very disturbed children and adolescents must work out his/her own personal checkpoints about the countertransference caused by the patient's or parent's mechanism of projective identification. I am not asserting that the specific theoretical perspectives I am recommending will be useful for every child and adolescent psychoanalyst; however, I do believe that without clear theoretical guidelines for working with severely disturbed parents, the unprepared psychoanalyst may feel that the situation has dramatically changed from treading water to suddenly drowning in very choppy waters and thinking that life could be much easier if one were to just see adults rather than crazy kids with their crazy parents.

Clinical Case Illustration #2

This clinical illustration considers a regularly recurring problem in dealing with parents: parental competitive envy. Parents frequently need to destroy the psychoanalyst's or therapist's efforts because of their unresolved feelings of envy, the feelings of envy aroused by the child's or adolescent's clinical improvement, or–most commonly–some combination of the above.

Lorie, a 3 year old Hispanic girl who was pulling out her hair, was referred to me as a low fee control [supervised] clinic case for a psychoanalysis by a psychoanalytic colleague. He was treating her mother, a single parent, privately in a 2x per week psychotherapy. From the moment Lorie entered my office until each session concluded, she was extremely animated with one school scene after another being enacted. She invariably assumed the role of the admonishing teacher and I was assigned the role of the hapless, pre-kindergarten student who was painfully learning how to behave to avoid the teacher's wrath. At the end of a session when Lorie's mother arrived early in the waiting room, Lorie did an about-face: she suddenly looked forlorn and depressed. I knew that this change of face was an important observation: however, I didn't grasp its significance for quite a long time.

For two years things went relatively smoothly during the once every six weeks or so meetings that I had scheduled with Lorie's mother. Although she impressed me as being up-tight and not very trusting, in general Lorie's mother was cooperative and friendly except for one occasion where I found myself suddenly enraged. She caught me off guard with her comment that her psychoanalyst had [gratuitously] told her that I was an inexperienced student who was experimenting on her daughter. I tried to respond in a non-defensive way by clarifying what I assumed to be her distortion and anxiety about supervised control cases.

About three months after this incident, I had moved my office to a newly constructed building conveniently located in downtown Chicago. Lorie's mother was initially very impressed with the location of my new office, the special play area for children, and the efficiency of the modern elevators. I was completely taken by surprise when one day she exploded into my office and expressed her outrage that I was risking her daughter's life because of the dangerous traffic near the entrance to my building. I found myself boiling inside; nevertheless, with a relatively calm exterior I explained that there were at least three ways that she and Lorie could reach my office without going anywhere near the building's parking lot. Since she didn't drive, I couldn't help asking myself: what was her problem? A few weeks later, she called for an appointment and answered my question.

Lorie's mother began this interview as if she had just discovered a secret affair. "You know she's in love with you, don't you know!" she screamed. "Lorie is much more clever than you think!" She then lamented that she was only seeing her doctor now once a week whereas Lorie was seeing me four times weekly. "It just isn't fair!" I said something about the possibility that there was an unconscious resonance from her own psychological past with Lorie's analysis which she might want to take up in her own treatment.

Lorie's mother was a deeply envious woman. She coveted the attention she saw Lorie getting in coming four times weekly and enviously felt herself to be shortchanged because her psychoanalyst, in her view, was withholding, and would only see her in a once per week psychotherapy. Her irrational attack about the dangerous traffic was the first indication of her need to destroy her daughter's treatment with me [unless there is some credibility to my speculative conjecture that perhaps she had somehow provoked her analyst's gratuitous attack on me]. I valued Lorie's mother's [correct] comment that I hadn't realized how clever Lorie was. I flashed to the waiting room scene and now it seemed perfectly clear: Lorie had grown up with an awareness that her mother was as deprived as she was. [This conjecture was supported 12 years later when Lorie and her mother returned to Chicago for an extended weekend and visited me in my office. I was struck by the role reversal: ''Hi Dr. Richmond,'' Lorie smiled. ''You remember my mother . . . and she placed her arm protectively around her mother's shoulder.] In the waiting room scene early in her analysis, Lorie had demonstrated her cleverness by trying to conceal from her mother her enjoyment of the sessions with me. She was doing her best to conceal her emotional attachment to me; her waif-like forlorn appearance underscored [among other meanings] that there was no benefit from her treatment that her mother would need to destroy. Since parental self esteem is naturally wounded when the psychoanalyst is perceived as being successful and the parent feels that he/she has failed, it is crucial to be vigilant in searching for indications of parental envy in working with disturbed children and adolescents.

Both of these clinical case illustrations demonstrate hidden counter-identification reactions which the psychoanalyst did not know how to process when they occurred. They also provide striking examples of the destructive narcissism (Rosenfeld) that becomes manifest when the parent regressively retreats to the psychological operations of the psychotic paranoid personality (Bion). These (schematic) clinical cases cogently demonstrate the need for a reliable theoretical model of the parental alliance and its vicissitudes. In general, we know how progressive and regressive processes operate to influence development. Perhaps the intensity of the different disruptions we experience in working with severely disturbed parents provides our best clue for understanding their disturbing psychopathology. A recent paper (Grand, S. et al., 1988) provides a useful classification of the levels of integrative failure seen with severe psychopathology. Their work could, I believe, further clarify the pioneering work of Bion, Rosenfeld, Searles and others whose observations and formulations have provided us with a conceptual language about severe psychopathology.

We know very little about how parental alliances form, develop and are sustained in severely disturbed parents with predominantly (paranoid) psychotic personalities. We know far more about how their destructive rage, competitive envy and projective identification mechanism may frequently disrupt the therapeutic process. With severely disturbed children and adolescents the absence of the patient's content requires the skilled processing of the analyst's counter-identification. Where there is paucity of content, counter-transference tensions become of paramount importance for clarifying and understanding the therapeutic process.

Clinical Case Illustration #3

With Sarah, a nineteen year old daughter of a wealthy business-man and schoolteacher wife, the profound archaic identification with her father combined with her distorted transference projections resulted in a very problematic therapeutic alliance. Matters were made considerably worse by various disruptive attempts by her parents who unabashedly set out to destroy the treatment. Disparaging remarks made directly to me about my competence at times led to severe self questioning and self-doubt (which Bion described as the destroying of linking). I gradually was able to perceive the intense negative therapeutic reaction that corresponded to whatever advances occurred during my sessions with Sarah. I gradually concluded that my interventions interfered with the parents' destructive process. (She had two other siblings who were dysfunctional. One had made a suicide attempt while the other required long term hospitalization.)

On one occasion, following the use of a narcotic agent, Sarah almost died. Since I had no idea of her drug abuse at that time and realized that Sarah could not share what she was experiencing with me, I insisted that she be hospitalized. Her mother became enraged and accused me of "pushing her buttons" to agitate her and her husband. I was accused of destroying the marriage and disrupting the family because of the tensions that I created by this recommendation. I suggested that an independent consultant be called. [I had already consulted privately with another senior colleague who had a great deal of experience with suicidal patients. He recommended hospitalization because he considered Sarah to be the kind of patient who would not be able to communicate in an honest way what she was experiencing.]

Several months later after Sarah returned from the hospital and resumed treatment with me, she acknowledged that it was not possible for her to cooperate with me. She explained to me that since her father hated doctors, so did she. Intellectually, she was very identified with his political, religious, and moral views. She thought I was OK–at times, but most of the time she thought of me as her persecutor. She never felt that she had an obligation to be truthful. When I suggested that there were times she misunderstood my intentions because of the way she viewed me, she initially disagreed. Eventually, Sarah grasped the reasons behind her fears which were related primarily to her destructive fantasies and archaic grandiosity. She resented every session: nevertheless, she called me once, spontaneously, for an emergency appointment after she had become convinced that she might actually kill her mother. "Get me out of there," she implored, "or I'll really go crazy."

Whenever I tried to talk to Sarah about her identification with her father, she resented the implication that she was not her own person; however, she gradually agreed that there were times when she was identifying with him. Sarah never acknowledged that he terrified her: however, as the treatment continued, she would imitate his foibles, mock his behavior, and criticize his political views.

Along with the helpless dependency and deep envy described in the first two clinical case illustrations, Sarah evidences many qualities consistent with Bion's depiction of schizoidal, (paranoid) psychotic character psychopathology. What impressed me most was the way her archaic merger/identification with her father [identification with the aggressor] left her secluded in her cocoon of schizoidal withdrawal with overly perfectionistic grandiose illusions of self sufficiency.

I found myself somewhat reluctant to recall the various countertransferences I experienced with Sarah and her parents. I found myself needing to consult about what was being stirred up in me with various colleagues (whom I carefully rotated so they wouldn't grasp how troubling Sarah was for me). At times the evoked countertransference seemed embarrassingly obvious, e.g., on one occasion her mother, who was being treated by a colleague, called me repeatedly while I was in the middle of a session with another patient. I indicated that I could not talk to her; however, if she wished, I could call her back at the end of the session and arrange a time to talk with her. An awkward silence ensued. Finally, I said in as sensitive a tone as I could muster: "I'm sorry but I am going to have to hang up." Later, I was berated by her (and questioned by her analyst) for doing the unthinkable: no one had ever hung up on her before. That weekend I found myself suffering from a terrible headache which persisted for about 36 hours. It abated rather quickly when I finally had the simple thought: "I really would like to murder Sarah's mother."

Countertransference: Pro et Contra

In contemporary psychoanalytic thinking the psychoanalyst's use of countertransference to clarify the therapeutic process is controversial. This stems in part from the original Reik-Reich debate in which Theodore Reik argued that the psychoanalyst's countertransferences could be useful in understanding the patient. He contended that the presence of countertransference does not necessarily mean that the psychoanalyst's analysis was incomplete. Wilhelm Reich, in opposing this view, stressed that if countertransferences occurred, it was necessary for the psychoanalyst to engage in self-analysis or seek additional analysis. Today, many analysts contend that those who emphasize the value of "countertransference analysis" run the dual risk of promoting idiosyncratic thinking and de-emphasizing the importance of the patient's clinical content from a process viewpoint. As a result of this controversy, the contributions of the British School of psychoanalytic authors, e.g., Donald Winnicott, Winnifred Bion and Herbert Rosenfeld, are still not accepted by Structural theory analysts and Self psychologists who oppose Kleinian/Object relations theory. This is unfortunate since, as I have emphasized, it is essential to use the countertransferences evoked by severely disturbed children, adolescents and their parents to overcome the inevitable impasses that result from their transferences.

Since the 1950's, an extensive [primarily Kleinian] literature on the use of countertransference developed. After Paula Heimann's 1960 paper (pp. 9-10), the role of countertransference for therapeutic technique took an irreversible, giant step forward. The British school of Object Relations theorists, following Heimann's lead, emphasized the value of the analyst learning [emotionally] how to sustain and deal with his/her countertransference feelings, rather than formulating interpretations predominantly based on schematic (intellectual) techniques.

For many classical psychoanalysts, the latter criticism remains a serious concern about modern self psychology. Critics believe that its current emphasis on the interpretation of the selfobject transference (without equal attention being given to the vicissitudes and degree of integration of the self's grandiose fantasy) results in an overly schematic, non-analytic psychotherapeutic process that is insufficient to work through unresolved (unconscious) narcissistic transferences. Those self-psychologists who do give equal attention to the vicissitudes of the patient's grandiose fantasy would argue that the narcissistic transferences can only be properly analyzed by the transference expansion of the patient's grandiose fantasy to assure that a meaningful analysis of the therapeutic process is continued. The critical question about the therapeutic efficacy of the structural theory approach to interpretive activity is whether there is increased accessibility to the patient's unconscious fantasy as opposed to an increase in the patient's unconscious resistance (Arlow, 1985).

These differences in thinking about the analyst's involvement with the patient has stirred great controversy both theoretically and clinically. In my view, the Kleinian viewpoint elaborated by Bion, Rosenfeld and the British school of Object Relations theorists does not necessarily improve matters in working with neurotic and narcissistic transferences; however, it does provide a better way to understand psychotic transferences involving projective identification.

TRANSFERENCE AND PROJECTIVE IDENTIFICATION

In diagnosing the transference with this group of children, adolescents and parents, it is necessary to clarify the interrelationship between transference, projective identification and countertransference.

Transference

Despite theoretical disputes about what constitutes transference, Freud's (1900) topographical model continues to be useful in explaining transference as an intrapsychic phenomenon. In neurotic and narcissistic transferences, the patient's unconscious object or self representations and their affective/drive components are transferred across the repression barrier onto preconscious object representations resulting in an intrapsychic, composite transference representation.

From the perspective of the self and object representational world, transference indicates a distortion of reality–the reality of the object world. Neurotic and psychotic transferences can be differentiated by the degree and quality of the distortion of reality that occurs.

Projective Identification

Before trying to clarify the concept of projective identification, it is useful to differentiate three interrelated intrapsychic mechanisms: projection, transference and displacement. In one usage of these terms, projection involves the attribution of part of a self representation to an object representation, whereas displacement involves the attribution of part of one object representation to another object representation (that is clearly differentiated from self representations). Our current conceptual language often includes the linking of transference with displacement.

The process of projective identification (Goldstein, W. 1991) is an integral component of the psychotic transferences of seriously disturbed parents (and patients) and elicits corresponding countertransference reactions. In contrast, the projections in neurotic and narcissistic transferences do not show this blurring of ego boundaries, nor is there evidence of the splitting processes that lead to projective identification.

A key component of projective identification is the mechanism of splitting. Melanie Klein first emphasized the importance of this concept (1946) which was further elaborated by both the British school and Otto Kernberg (1967). Some patients overuse splitting –

– (vs. repression) from earliest infancy and then continue to use this
– mechanism as a defence vs. conflict (Segal, H. 1990). Splitting is
a necessary precursor for initiating the process of projective identification.

When projective identification is instigated as a result of the
splitting mechanism, self and object representations are blurred
because, intrapsychically, parts of the self are split off from the
remaining self and projected onto the object representation. This
part of the process leads to an identification with the object; however,
the form of identification differs significantly from the processes
involved in neurotic identifications. Recently, Thomas Ogden
(1986) has formulated a model of the sequence of steps that constitutes what might be described as the complete process of projective
identification and which accounts for the psychoanalyst's countertransference of feeling pressured to think, feel, and act in accor-
dance with the patient's projection.

As I have stated, it is useful to think of projective identification
as an integral part of the psychotic transference [Bion] which is
seen (predominantly) in seriously disturbed individuals. Most analysts agree with the distinction between projection and the more
primitive mechanism of projective identification; however, they do
not believe that the latter is exclusively a psychotic mechanism.

Countertransference/Counteridentification

To understand the countertransference experience due to projective identification when trying to deal effectively with parents
who behave in a disorganizing or disruptive manner, it is essential
to recognize the blurring of the parent's disorganized self representation with his/her disorganized object representation.

The emphasis in this paper on the counteridentification type of
countertransference requires some explanation. In advocating the
value of processing the psychoanalyst's counteridentification as a
– potential organizer to clarify the patient's transference, I am trying
→to make a distinction between two forms of empathic closure. The
empathic vicarious introspection recommended by Kohut (in contrast to clinical intuition) requires a sound knowledge of one's own
childhood neurotic conflictual themes and narcissistic tensions.
During a session or a sequence of therapeutic hours a psychological

theme or repeated pattern may emerge in which one can transiently identify with the child's or adolescent's anxiety, guilt, boredom, etc., and use this insight to formulate the therapeutic process. Although Kohut (1968, 1971, 1977) wrote about the inherent difficulties in dealing with the various countertransferences evoked by narcissistic transferences, he neglected the connection between more severe pathological forms of narcissism and paranoid processes. The second form of empathic closure occurs when the psychoanalyst processes the countertransference counteridentification that results from the impact of the patient's or parent's projective identification mechanism.

In using the term countertransference-counteridentification I knowingly am blurring the distinction between transference and resistance; however, my purpose in doing so is to emphasize the differences in the clinical experiences that lead to these two forms of empathic closure. Ralph Greenson (1960) was so convinced of the value of empathic constructions that occurred against the analyst's internal resistance that he preferred to reserve the term empathy for these integrations of the patient's clinical material. What other analysts referred to as empathic closure was, for Greenson, either ordinary sensitivity or clinical intuition derived from broadly based clinical experience.

CONCLUSION

This paper with its emphasis on counteridentification responses to projective identification is intended to provide an introduction to the significant role that the psychoanalyst's countertransference may play in clarifying the therapeutic process with very disturbed children, adolescents and their parents.

BIBLIOGRAPHY

Abrams, S. (1977) "The Genetic Point of View: Historical Antecedents and Developmental Transformations" New York: Journal of the American Psychoanalytic Association 25:417-426.
Arlow, Jacob (1985) Panel, American Psychoanalytic Association, Fall Meeting.
Bernstein, Haskell (1990) Being Human. New York: Gardner Press Inc.

Freud, S. (1900) The Interpretation of Dreams. London: The Hogarth Press Standard Edition Volume V 610-622.

Grand, S., Freedman, N., Feiner, K., and Kiersky, S. (1988) "Notes on the Progressive and Regressive Shifts in Levels of Integrative Failure: A Preliminary Report on the Classification of Severe Psychopathology" Madison, Conn.: Psychoanalysis and Contemporary Thought 11: #4 :705-740.

Goldstein, W. (1991) An Introduction to the Borderline Conditions. Northvale, New Jersey: Jason Aronson, Inc.

Greenson, R. (1960) "Empathy and its Vicissitudes" London: International Journal of Psychoanalysis 41:418-424.

Grinberg, L., Sor, D., and Tabak de Bianchedi, E. (1977) Introduction to the Work of Bion. New York: Jason Aronson, Inc.

Heimann, Paula (1960) "Counter-transference" London: British Journal of Medical Psychology 33: 9-15.

Kernberg, O. (1967) "Borderline Personality Organization" New York: Journal of the American Psychoanalytic Association 15: 641-685.

Klein, M. (1946) "Notes on some Schizoid Mechanisms" London: International Journal of Psychoanalysis 26:11-33.

Kohut, H. (1966) "Forms and Transformations of Narcissism" New York: Journal of the American Psychoanalytic Association 14:243-272.

Kohut, H (1971) The Analysis of the Self. New York: International Universities Press.

Kohut, H. (1977) The Restoration of the Self. New York: International Universities Press.

Modell, A. (1990) "The psychoanalytic setting as a container of multiple levels of reality: A perspective on the theory of psychoanalytic treatment." Hillsdale, New Jersey: Psychoanalytic Inquiry 9:67-87.

Modell, A. (1990) Other Times, Other Realities. Cambridge, Massachusetts: Harvard University Press.

Ogden, T. (1990) The Matrix of the Mind. Northvale, New Jersey: Jason Aronson, Inc.

Rosenfeld, H. (1987) Impasse and Interpretation. London: The New Library of Psychoanalysis.

Segal, H. (1990) Panel, American Psychoanalytic Association, Fall Meeting.

Everything to Help, Nothing to Hinder: Grandiosity, Ambivalence and Boundaries in the Parent-School Alliance

Daniel Frank, PhD

INTRODUCTION

There's a well known story from the lore of Jewish mysticism. A student had been working very hard to understand a passage of text. After many long hours of study, he felt he was ready to show his teacher, a learned rabbi, what he had learned. With excitement and fear he approached his teacher. The teacher listened as the student spoke. When the student finished his explanation, the teacher paused. "You have done well," the teacher said. "You have understood the meaning of the black ink that is written on the page. Now go and tell me the meaning of the white spaces which surround the black print."

Presence and absence.

What we see and what is hidden from easy sight.

Psychoanalysis teaches us about presence and absence; about manifest and latent content; about conscious, preconscious and unconscious meanings; about what we feel, what we reveal and what we conceal about ourselves; about how silence can communicate something vital and real, and how talk can cloud and confuse genuine communication, and how clouded talk can express genuine ambivalent feeling.

Presence and absence.

What we remember and what we forget.

We are what we remember and we are what we forget.

So let us not forget that history is what we think about the past; that community is comprised of a past we continue to share in the present; that there is indeed an important institutional history to our collaborative work with children and their families: Bruno Bettelheim came to Chicago, and ultimately to the Orthogenic School of the University of Chicago, to work with Ralph Tyler, long time professor here at the University and former board member of the Institute for Psychoanalysis, when Dr. Tyler was project director of the landmark Eight Year Study which involved research and study of the Francis W. Parker School.

Presence and absence.

What we remember and what we forget.

Who we remember and who we cannot forget.

Zanvel Klein, child psychologist, teacher, scholar, and participant in this institutional history, understood the dynamics of presence and absence in the lives of troubled children and his recent death will remain a loss to all of us who knew him.

The title of my paper is: "Everything to Help, Nothing to Hinder: Grandiosity, Ambivalence and Boundaries in the Parent-School Alliance."[1]

In this paper, I will convey how psychoanalytic concepts and psychoanalysis as a method of inquiry can help us understand the variety of ways parents and schools can experience each other, especially when they meet to discuss the welfare of a troubled child.

The paper has four sections:

1. An opening section on the problems involved in forming a positive alliance.
2. A section in which I discuss the dynamics of idealization.
3. A section in which I discuss the vicissitudes of disillusionment.
4. A section on the rhythms of reparation in the parent-school alliance.

THE PROBLEM OF ALLIANCE

All schools have cultures, and all cultures have values, beliefs and practices which give its members a sense of belonging and identification. The meanings these practices and beliefs have for its members contribute significantly to the formation of a coherent sense of who they are as persons in that community.

In the school I attended as a boy—and in which I now work as an adult—the school's philosophy of education and tradition of learning guide students, teachers and parents as each tries to find his or her own place in the life of the school. All human action—hallway conversations, classroom lessons, athletic competition, dramatic and artistic performances, and official school policies—are assessed in light of the school's dominant cultural beliefs.

It is not unusual, for example, for students, teachers, parents and administrators to refer, at various times and for a variety of reasons, to the school's well-respected code of oral and written tradition. Dialogue of this kind happens throughout the school—in hallways, playgrounds, classrooms, locker rooms, and, of course, at formal school functions. The code is open and accessible to all. Each member of the school community is entitled, indeed encouraged, to interpret the meaning of events in the cultural life of the school. This practice gives people a sense of heritage, permanence and authority. It gives them the meaningful feeling that, as much as any one else in the school, each individual can lay authoritative claim to understanding the life of the school. This participatory practice gives the school a vital sense of social coherence through its allegiance to the school's founding democratic ideals.

A favorite, and easy to remember line, even for the younger students, is: "Everything to help and nothing to hinder." First said nearly ninety years ago by Colonel Francis Wayland Parker, the late nineteenth century educator, father of progressive education, once Civil War solider, colleague of the University of Chicago's John Dewey, and founder of the school which bares his name on Chicago's north side, this line has balance and beauty in its style and symmetry: everything and nothing; help or hindrance; the certainty of either/or. It also suggests more than a pinch of grandiosity.

As a child, I remember having heard this phrase along with such words as "community," "responsibility," "model home," and "embryonic democracy." I also remember seeing this phrase printed on the postmark of letters my parents received from the school. I remember how we students liked this phrase. We felt it meant that the teachers really cared about us. The ideal expressed in these words–"Everything to help and nothing to hinder," made us feel wanted, worthy, indeed, entitled to have our needs met by the adults in our lives–at least our needs as we thought we understood them at the time. The presence of that almost battle-cry phrase in the language of the school's culture made us feel supported; that the school was indeed *our* school, our home away from home, our world. This ideal, expressed in hyperbole, had the ring of the absolute, the sound of profound certainty, an open invitation to a sense of mission. It gave us the sense that somehow the world would give us the benefit of the doubt.

And that is what schools should do. Beyond the job of teaching students basic language and computational skills, schools have the opportunity to contribute to the development of a student's sense of self as a capable, critical and creative learner. A child's experience in school can support the development of a solidifying self-image; that of a worthwhile person, liked by teachers and able to make friends and produce good work in a way which affirms rather than depletes self-esteem. Schools have the potential not only to make students believe that their efforts should contribute to the good of humanity but also that they have developed the talent to realize this goal and feel that their own concrete contributions can actually make a difference. Schools should have this kind of positive influence in children's lives. After all, second only to their own families, children spend more time in school than in any other social institution.

"Everything to help and nothing to hinder." These simple words, less than a hundred years old, capture the spirit of a story more than two thousand years-old and provide an opening into the problem of how we, as educators, clinicians and parents, struggle to understand the complexity of human experience and the meaning of human relationships.

The story goes: A wise guy once approached the revered teacher, Rabbi Hillel. The man challenged the rabbi to explain the whole of Torah, the whole of Judaism, while he would stand on one foot. The man shifted his weight. With a foot in the air, the wise guy listened to the wise man say: "Do not do to others what you would not have them do to you." The rabbi paused. The cynic was about to lose his balance as the sage added, "All the rest is commentary."

For me, it was a high school shop teacher who clued me in to the complicated world of measured interpretation, philosophical agility and moral consistency. A student was trying to talk his way out of class early but our teacher would not let him, saying, instead, that the student needed to complete the task to which he had already committed himself. In classic adolescent fashion, the student reached for his ace-in-the-hole. "C'mon man, let me go early. You know, 'Everything to help and nothing to hinder.'" The teacher paused. I can see the student shift his weight. "Sometimes," the teacher said to the student, "'Everything to help and nothing to hinder' means saying 'yes,' and sometimes it means saying, 'no.'"

And there it was. One phrase, one guiding ideal and two different interpretations, two different and incompatible points of view. Help was experienced as hindrance; and hindrance was experienced as no help at all.

Those of us who work with children and their parents confront this problem in our daily practice, whether it is in a school, a clinician's office or other settings. Clinicians, for example, must think about issues of "yes" and "no" all the time as they consider the therapeutic effects of abstinence, gratification and neutrality in the management of their relationships to patients. What kind of interventions are helpful, what kind might be experienced as harmful? How does the patient experience the timing, content and tone of an interpretation?

A patient and therapist can see the world in very different ways. A therapist's interpretation can be offered to help a patient gain insight; the patient, however, can experience the therapist's interpretation as a pain in the neck, the will of somebody else's agenda, a refusal to satisfy some very deep wishes. World views apart, a patient pushes for desire; a therapist for understanding.

In one way or another, we each hold the phrase, "Everything to help and nothing to hinder," as a guiding ideal. In one way or another, we also have to understand how to apply this concept in the specific contexts of each child and each family. This is especially true in those cases where children seem to be suffering from more than their fair share of troubles.

For most children, school stands midway between home and community. Schools provide children with the potential for a transitional space between a child's experience of family values and expectations and the child's own emerging sense of the values and expectations held by the wider society. In their socially sanctioned role, schools perform a public mandate, a cultural function, indeed a moral mission, to help parents prepare children for lives as autonomous adults capable of contributing as responsible citizens to the welfare of the broader community. When successful, schools are able to support, complement, supplement and compensate for a child's experience of his or her own family and neighborhood.

A child's school experience is supported in profoundly important ways when parents, teachers, counselors, advisors and administrators are working together on the child's behalf. This is especially true for children who are experiencing significant academic, social and emotional problems. When parents, and the schools which their children attend, are able to develop a positive, collaborative working relationship, the children's best interests can be addressed. For the care and education of those children who are having serious difficulty learning in school or managing to feel good about their relationships with teachers, schoolmates or family members, it is especially important for schools and parents to perceive each other as allies who can talk to each other as they work toward a common goal.

This is the ideal. This is what we aim for. This is what we know to be right.

But let's not forget that Freud suggested that education, along with government and psychoanalysis, is an impossible profession. There are many factors–social, economic, cultural, political and psychological–which actively impede the development of a trusting alliance between parents and schools.

In our nation's urban public schools, parents, teachers and administrators fight huge odds. They fight oppression, incompetence, and $350 million deficits. They fight our national history, an economy which punishes the poor, union interests and downtown city hall politics. For too many American children, education is made all but impossible as entrenched poverty, neglect and violence have made schools dangerous and frightening places to learn and teach. For too many, the promise of a nurturing "holding environment" (Winnicott, 1965) for learning and psychological growth has been out muscled by the seething despair of an underclass strangle-holding environment. For too many, schools actively contribute to their feelings of emptiness, rage and loss.

On the other side of town, private schools are removed, for the most part, from the desperation and futility felt by so many whose lives are affected by life in inner city public schools. Yet, even in these more exclusive and less chaotic institutions, children and families experience their own social and psychological troubles which affect the ways in which parents and schools struggle to develop positive working relationships. Even in these schools, which promote a public presentation of warm, family-like relationships, different personal histories and different roles tend to promote different world views and competing interpretations about what parents and the school need to do in order to be helpful to children, especially troubled children. Cooperation and competition are both integral aspects of human relationships present in all societies. And yet it is especially difficult in schools which pride themselves on good will, cooperative spirit and a shared sense of democratic citizenship to recognize and acknowledge the presence of hostile and aggressive feelings toward fellow community members: colleagues, students and parents. Schools and parents are necessary partners in the life of a child. The relationship is a logical one. As in any relationship, however, the parent-school relationship is vulnerable to irrational responses shaped from the transferences each party brings to their encounters with the other. Parents send more than their children to school, and teachers and administrators bring more to work than their briefcases. Each is also accompanied by his or her own memories and associations to their own childhood school and family experiences.

We have all been to school. We all have memories of our childhood and adolescent days as students. A teacher, a classroom, some classmates, an assignment well done, a test failed, a good deed, a mischievous act. Stories of all kinds. Parents and teachers alike bring with them to current school situations their own fantasies and associations to past school experiences. These fantasies include feelings of longing and revenge; the desire for reparation and mastery over past psychological wounds, and the desire for immortality through reliving what now seems like once simpler days, now long gone to the complexities of adult life and the middle-aged realization that, as adults, they have probably already lived most of their lives. These memories and associations can, unwittingly, influence the here-and-now formation of a parent-school alliance.

Michael Basch has reminded us that, "It is the management of the transferences that people have toward us as authorities and/or helpers (and one's reaction to them) that determines how successful both teachers and psychoanalysts will ultimately be in carrying out their respective tasks (1989:773)." The management of the transferences are complicated by the dynamics of grandiosity, narcissism, ambivalence, persecution and reparation. These dynamics affect the ways in which schools and parents perceive themselves and each other. These issues indeed complicate and characterize most parent-school relationships. Awareness of how these dynamics affect the parent-school alliance can mean the difference between hope and despair in the life of a family. The management of the parent-school relationship needs to develop in a way which does not jeopardize an essential sense of physical and psychological safety. For parents and school representatives to discuss with each other, even cautiously, the range of options which are in the best interests of a child who is experiencing significant troubles, both parties need to feel they are working in a reliable and consistent environment of trusted protective care. In this manner; the "good enough school" must find ways to manage the inevitable idealizations, disillusionments and conflicts which will arise when working with parents.

IDEALIZATION, THE SCHOOL AND THE PARENT

The school can and should offer itself to families as an idealized and idealizable object. Aspects of grandiosity can be very beneficial as parents and children need to feel that their educational needs are being addressed in a steady, dependable and even masterful manner. The identifications established with the school's philosophy help parents solidify a coherent sense of good feeling about themselves as they feel connected to an ideal larger than themselves. In this way, the school can serve as a dependable guiding parental figure to its families.

In this transference, old patterns of relating to school persist. Parents want to be good. They want to like teachers and they want to be liked by their children's teachers. They don't want to feel that they have done something wrong and thus may jeopardize the teacher's good feeling toward them. Even highly competent, successful and powerful men and women, can feel anxious and intimidated when a teacher or administrator calls them to talk about a matter concerning their child. They feel as if they themselves had done something wrong; as if they were back in school and were being sent to the principal's office.

Parents display these feelings through an enactment of a variety of transferences. Some parents are extremely compliant, even solicitous. Others can be extremely provocative and challenging in their efforts to show the school and themselves that they are doing the right thing for their children. This tendency is natural, expected and, as we know, psychologically complicated. Behavior can belie questions: Do you like my children? Do you think I am a good parent? Do you like me?

Parents want to feel that they are helping their children and meeting their needs. Particularly, and appropriately, they want to feel that they have done the right thing by having chosen the school as a good enough partner with whom they can share the responsibility of raising and caring for their children. This feeling is heightened when parents are paying substantial sums in tuition. Competition for admission to a private school can be stiff, and, with few inner city options available, parents can become desperate to find refuge from the public school system. Almost frantic for shelter, parents are indeed ripe for wishing the school to be great, powerfully competent and unendingly resourceful and caring for their children. In this way, admission to a private school can be experienced by parents as an act of protection and care . . . aided perhaps by the fortune of good luck and the hand of God. For these parents, what makes education an impossible profession is the slim chance of having a child admitted to a private school and then being able to pay the ever-rising tuition to keep their child in the school. In this context, parents can also feel that a private school education–almost independent of their child's own academic success–is a sign of self-validation; a sign of their own importance, competence and achievement.

A school can join a parent's fantasy in several ways. The school can set ideals of high expectations and grandiose claims about what it can accomplish with its students. The school can claim it teaches the "whole child," not just a part. It can claim it teaches for more than excellence; it can claim it educates for character. It can claim it does more than prepare students for college; it can claim it prepares them for life. It can claim it does more than teach fundamental communication and computational skills; it can claim it builds self-esteem and the courage to take meaningful risks. It can claim it does more than nurture the growth and development of each individual student; it can claim it develops within each student a deep and lasting sense of care and commitment to the common social good.

Moreover, the school can ask parents to care about their child's education in the same way the school does. It can state that parents should believe in the school's philosophy in the same way that teachers and alumni do. It can claim the moral authority to expect parents to join their children and become involved as active volunteers in the life of the school.

The school and the parent each need to feel appreciated by the other. Each needs to see in the face of the other a warm, appreciating, even loving, glow. Parents want to feel they are being good parents; teachers want to feel they are doing a good job. For a variety of reasons, each party can feel uneasy and doubtful about their own competence in the roles they assume. Pointing to the state of our nation's public schools and to the growing numbers of children who grow up poor in our country, many educators believe that children are not especially valued in our culture. Accordingly, they argue, adults who work with children are not afforded much meaningful social status. Consequently, teachers can feel uneasy and vulnerable about their own self-esteem when working with wealthy, powerful parents, who in their own right, can have their own grandiose notions about themselves and their children's capabilities.

Yet, as long as parents feel the school is living up to their wished for perceptions of the school as a place where promises are kept and needs are cared for, the school will continue to be idealized. And as long as the school feels parents appreciate its efforts to care for and educate their children, the school can maintain itself as an idealizable figure in the lives of families.

Things are fine as long as things are fine.

But what happens when something goes wrong? What happens to the parent-school relationship when a child develops problems and is having difficulty thriving in the school? How does the alliance experience the events which lead teachers and counselors to talk about a student's problems, or parents complain about the difficulty their child is having in a teacher's classroom? What feelings are evoked when parents, teachers and administrators talk about matters impeding a child's successful growth and progress? How does this inquiry affect the psychological balance of adult narcissism and self-esteem?

DISILLUSIONMENT, LOSS AND AMBIVALENCE

Schooling is an emotionally charged business. Perhaps more than any other enterprise, schools are charged with the care of parents' often most cherished and precious connection to life: their children as representations of themselves; as representations of their own unique sense of self. In this context, children are not their own persons. A student in a classroom is not simply a student in a chair, at a desk, taking notes, passing notes or staring out the window. That young person exists, in some form, as an extension of all that has gone right and all that has gone wrong in his or her parents' lives. A student's school experience can represent parental anxieties about success and failure as well as generations of family hopes and dreams for a better future. And that is not all. A student in a classroom is also likely to serve as a reflection of the teacher's own sense of competence as a professional and as a person. Independent of each individual parent and teacher's own unique personality, there exists a normative psychological climate in which students, parents, teachers and administrators are likely to experience each other as persons who either help or hinder the maintenance of his or her own self-esteem.

Children can make parents feel acutely vulnerable. When the

school begins to question a child's functioning, parents can easily take matters painfully to heart. Inquiry into our children's actions can make us feel anxious and ambivalent. In these inquiries, we tell stories and make interpretations. Our accounts portray our desire to challenge and respond as well as our fear of risk and the unknown. Our constructions demonstrate our ability to retain balance and lose our footing. In our statements, and in what we hear of other people's statements, we struggle with the tendency to reveal and to conceal. What we ask and what we question betray our wish to know and our wish not to know. In the same single moment, we can seek knowledge and understanding and we can tenaciously subvert that very search.

For example, parents can appreciate the school's interest and attention given to their child. Yet, parents also experience–in a heightened and exaggerated way–the school's inquiry as a criticism of their ability to raise children. And they can experience a call from a teacher, dean, counselor or principal as a rejection, as an abandonment by the school of its relationship to the family as a caring parental figure. In this regard, questions are perceived as an attack; inquiry as a form of persecution. In their anguish and distress, it becomes difficult, if only for a period of time, for parents to tolerate and manage ambivalent feelings; to balance their feelings of love and hate, appreciation and rage at the school.

These issues are heightened even more when the school is in the process of considering whether or not it will counsel a student out of the school. Despite–and because of–seemingly strong prior attachments to the school, talk of counseling out is almost always experienced by parents as a disruptive life event which leaves them feeling suddenly and unexpectedly traumatized and humiliated. Despite significant and methodical assessment, if the school feels it can no longer meet the child's developmental needs–and that it is in the best interest of the child to attend a different school–parents can nonetheless feel that the school is not living up to its claim of: "Everything to help and nothing to hinder." They feel they have been cruelly assaulted and heartlessly abandoned. They feel they have been ruthlessly betrayed.

The school, on the other hand, is likely to perceive its own actions as consistent with its philosophy. Even as staff might have to manage potential ambivalent and guilt feelings, the school would need to proceed with its assessment that to hold on to a student whose needs it can no longer meet would be irresponsible and hindering to the child's development. From this perspective, to counsel a student out would represent every effort on the part of the school to help parents understand the need to find an alternative educational setting which can more appropriately meet their child's needs.

Clearly, not all parents experience the school's inquiry as an attack. In many cases, parents are relieved to hear from the school. Parents may have had their own concerns about one of their children and may have felt additional anxiety when interpreting the school's silence as a sign that the school is either not observant, or that the school is not concerned enough about their child. As one parent said, "I'm so glad you called. We've been terribly worried. We just thought the school didn't care."

The school, at times, is no less vulnerable to feeling attacked by the presence of a question. "What is going on in that math class?" "Why did that teacher speak to my child that way?" "Who is in charge here, anyway?" Parental inquiry about a teacher's functioning or about an administrative decision has the potential to make school staff feel vulnerable and attacked, hurt and unappreciated. There is, in schools, a strong sense shared by staff, that we are the professionals, the educators. The curriculum is *our* domain. *We* are the authorities. "Don't ask us questions, don't tell us what to do," and, as the old line goes, "just drop your kid off the day after Labor Day and pick him up around the beginning of June." And yet, when pride and self-esteem are injured, powerful and ambivalent feelings can arise. School people want autonomy but they also can feel enraged when they think parents are not doing their job and instead are turning to the school to take on even more roles that were once reserved for the family, the physician or the church. In schools where parents are encouraged to participate in the life of the school, this contrary and ambivalent attitude poses some very real conflicts.

The roots of human ambivalence can be found in the early experience of our first relationships. One should not, therefore, be surprised to find that the anxiety of inquiry permeates the earliest moments in the school's relationship with a family. It can become no small concern to the school to know whether a family has sent their child to the school because of the parents' deep belief and allegiance to the school's philosophy or because the school was one of the very few alternatives to big city public education. A marriage of convenience, not a union of love. Their narcissism injured, their sense of specialness rejected, persons in the school can feel devalued, unappreciated, victimized. Unable to acknowledge their own rage at parents, school staff can project an image of parents as a hostile, unreasonable group, ready to take siege of the school, fire its faculty, change its philosophy, rewrite its very history, even give the school a new name.

These feelings represent fantasies organized around a social defense (Hirschhorn, 1988). Anxiety is contained by separating good from bad feelings and attributing one's own unacknowledged negative feelings to another group. This emotional configuration can inform the school's sometimes unwitting tendency to imagine parents as feeling hostile in routine evening parent meetings, individual parent conferences and, of course, on certain parent phone calls.

Recently, in the school where I work, a series of brightly colored, well-designed posters have appeared in the halls and other public places in the school. Printed in bold and appealing graphics, each of the nearly forty signs contain a different appealing black and white photograph of students and teachers engaged in learning and playing, and a different quotation culled from various students, teachers and parents associated with the school over its ninety year history. These quotations contribute to the dynamic feeling of life in the halls. In a visually appealing way, the posters add an important historical dimension to the fast pace of contemporary school life. They give us a sense that the work of today is connected to ideals of the past.

The project was conceived and designed by parents and staff associated with the school's Development Office. The idea for the project stemmed directly from the concern that too many current parents do not adequately understand the nature and mission of the school. The aim was to help promote a more effective way to educate parents about the values and philosophy of the school. But more to the point, the project's purpose was to respond to the school's feeling that its philosophy, its curriculum and its personnel–are not truly appreciated. Freud taught us how appearance disguises other dimensions of reality: the happy colors and lofty ideals now posted around the school are efforts to transform the darker feelings of injury, abandonment and powerlessness.

For these very reasons of vulnerable self-regard, and its manifested defenses, school staff can fall prey to avoiding calling a family when a student is experiencing marked difficulty. To call is to add one more case to one's busy and often overloaded schedule. To call is to come to terms with a full range of conflicting feeling about what it means to be caretaker. To call is to admit one's limitations; that one has failed in an heroic act and cannot care for the child alone. To call is to face the anxieties of letting go; of facing more directly possible lurking feelings of hostility and aggression toward the child, the family, and perhaps even colleagues in the school. To call is to acknowledge an elation of relief at having finally disposed of a long-term problem; and to call is to feel the guilt of failure and the humiliation of having to ask for help from an unconsciously perceived enemy. Who says schools aren't a part of the real world?

In a school with a tradition which claims to promote the development of student growth and autonomy in preparation for responsible adult citizenship in a democratic society, it is indeed intriguing to consider the ways in which parents and teachers–intelligent and accomplished people–can be psychologically prone to battle each other over unconscious claims to colonize the child's life with competing claims for being the child's true advocate, defender and savior. In this context, part of the trouble with the troubled child is the narcissism of the adults in his or her life.

TOWARD A REPARATIVE PROCESS

But just as there is the tendency in the human condition to project feared feelings onto others, there is also the corresponding tendency to seek healing and integration of split-off feelings. Reparation is as strong a force in human experience as is retaliation and revenge (Klein, 1936/1964). Each of us knows how life is complicated by its contradictions, how we can love and hate the same person at the same time. We know how it feels to be frazzled, overwhelmed, split; how it feels to live with ambivalence; and how that tension is part of what it means to be human. As individuals, each of us strives to balance the many different responsibilities and feelings we have. In this way, we are each trying to better integrate our own personal lives. In a world so often marked by uncertainty, disorder and disintegration, each of us nonetheless struggles to feel coherent, organized, whole. When we are able to acknowledge those painful feelings we have split-off and projected on to others, and instead retain those feelings in a more integrated and balanced manner, we have the opportunity to be better situated psychologically to understand another person's experience in a caring and empathic manner.

The problem with alliance is the problem of empathy. Only when we have been able to sustain a process of reparation within ourselves, can we provide the help others seek from us. Only when we can experience our own inquiries and the inquiries of others as efforts to understand and not as hostile attacks, can we develop the necessary perspective to offer parents and their troubled children the flexibility and firmness they need to aid them through difficult times.

In this light, teachers and administrators can be empathically aware of the ways in which many children experience their difficulties and troubles. In both public and private schools, teachers and administrators have been noticing how children's lives are becoming more complicated and affected by the labyrinth of choices and pressures their parents are experiencing. A consequence of these changing social demands has been that both public and private school teachers and administrators are feeling that families are increasingly turning to schools to take responsibility for areas of a child's life which had formerly been that of the family's (Welsh, 1987).

Schools have long played a central role in supporting the family, yet many educators are feeling that the boundaries between school and the family are shifting. Fundamental assumptions of role have altered. In the past, the school has supported the family as the central moral institution in a child's life. Now, the perception is, the school is being asked to play an equal, if not primary role, in the care and education of children. Many parents, feeling caught between the demands of their roles and/or the demands of their ambitions, are also feeling afraid to confront their own anger and aggression and their child's anger and aggression, and, consequently, want the school to play tough and be the heavy. In response to this request, teachers, counselors, deans and principals often can feel overburdened and resentful.

And yet, school people also understand how children all too often end up in the middle of adult disagreement and negotiation. As fathers and mothers are pulled by ambition and the demands of a leaner economy to put in long hours at work, the culture is placing increased demands on schools and children to manage themselves. Social reality has brought to too many children of high-tuition schools the psychological pains of divorce and hurried personal schedules. Too many of these children lead lives of highly organized after-school and weekend routines. As parents' lives become more complicated, they want their children to feel cared for in their absence. Consequently, parents seek to arrange their children's lives with activities they themselves believe are purposeful, productive and meaningful. Though these parents are well intended, many educators believe that children's lives are becoming more and more organized around parental anxieties to gain greater control over their own uneasiness about life's uncertainties. These observers of child and adolescent daily life continue to decry the perceived loss of free play time and the opportunity for adults to help children learn how to manage their own time. These children, often of separated or blended families, are the children of the hassled and harried pace, the children of lonely latchkey pseudo-autonomy, the child-objects of adult-centered "quality time" fantasies.

Schools need to respond empathically to the needs of these children. School people need to do "everything to help and nothing to hinder" a child's welfare, especially when the child may be experiencing significant difficulty in schoolwork, relationships with schoolmates, or at home.

We have come full circle: The rabbi, the Colonel and the shop teacher meet:

"Do not do to others what you would not have them do to
you."
"Everything to help and nothing to hinder."
"Sometimes that means saying 'yes'; sometimes that means
saying 'no.'"

What is help?
What is hindrance?

It has always been a matter of interpretation. Our relationships
with others are indeed constantly mediated by the vicissitudes
through which we interpret our relationship to the world around us.
The interpretations we make of our experience with others, imbed-
ded in the stories we tell about our lives, is how we hope to find
meaning in the things we say and do and hear and dream. Through
interpretation, we hope to explain to ourselves the ways in which
we feel connected and disconnected from others; the ways in which
we understand and misunderstand them, and ourselves; the ways in
which we, in turn, feel understood and misunderstood by others.
Through interpretation, and the narrative form those interpretations
take, we try to make sense of our lives.

In our efforts to understand the dynamics of the parent-school
relationship, we have seen how issues of grandiosity, ambivalence
and narcissism complicate and characterize the development of a
trusted parent-school alliance, creating a climate for competing
interpretations to emerge. Even in the best of schools, the best of
what civilization can offer its children, the force of human envy,
fear, rage and aggression finds its way on campus.

Schools may reach the conclusion that it is necessary to counsel
out a very troubled child. It may determine that this action is necessary and consistent with its interpretation of: "Everything to help
and nothing to hinder." Yet schools may also decide that each case
warrants its own approach.

A child who is having severe difficulty functioning in school
may have even more difficulty engaging in psychotherapy while the
school tries to work with parents through the emotional trauma and
the bureaucratic nightmare of securing state funds for residential
placement. As part of the treatment plan, the school and the therapist can agree to switch roles. The school, then, can become the

temporary holding environment for the child while the therapist struggles to engage the child in treatment.

A child who is several years behind classmates in reading comprehension and math skills can also be living through his or her parents' viciously contested divorce. Although the school can assess that it is not meeting the child's real academic needs, the school can, in collaboration with the child's therapist, decide, in the best interest of the child, to keep the child in school and wait out the storm of the divorce. The school, then, can provide the child with a stable and caring environment during a very turbulent time in the child's life. Later, after the worst of the divorce is over, and with no improvement in academic functioning, the school can then decide if and when it is time for the child to pursue education elsewhere. And even with this plan, the final stages of the counseling out process can be traumatic as the now divorced parents can still fight each other and the school every step of the way.

Once again: world views apart. Help can be experienced as hindrance and hindrance can be experienced as no help at all. Sometimes, no matter what the timing, informed interpretations are not well received.

In other cases, the school can tell a set of parents that their child needs to undergo a psychological evaluation if the school is going to be able to understand, and then assess the nature of the child's academic and social difficulties in the classroom. Some parents can be resistant to this idea. Several years of battling can ensue. In response to the resistance, the school can decide not to renew a child's contract for the coming year. Law suits can be threatened. And, later on, despite a difficult parting, parents can contact the school saying how much better their child is doing at a school for children with learning difficulties. They can express how grateful they are to the school for being firm in its position. Help can finally be interpreted as help. And, at other times, there are no happy endings. Schools can decide, despite all efforts to meet a child's needs, that it must counsel a student out. In these moments, separation can be experienced by all involved–the child, the parents, the school and the therapist–as a cruel scar of failure and sadness, a relationship gone awry, ruptured beyond repair.

One final note. Part of what is necessary in the reparative process of developing a positive working alliance with parents is that the school be aware of its need to be absolved from the guilt of letting a child go. The guilt feelings which accompany the off-time departure of a child from the school, can affect the teachers, counselors and administrators involved, and complicate the clear-headed decisions they have to make. In this sense, "Everything to help and nothing to hinder" means being able to acknowledge one's desire to want relief from the tension of our anxiety, our guilt, our shame, our conflicts, our deepest uncertainties, and the maturity to accept those feelings and live with the struggle to understand them.

NOTE

1. I want to acknowledge my appreciation to the following people for discussing their work and thoughts on this topic with me: John Cotton, Alice Ducas, Lil Lowry, Norma Nelson, Jan Sullivan, Robert Koff, M.D., Carol Levine Frank, Paul Gedo, Ph.D., and Merylin Salomon, Ph.D. The responsibility for the formulations presented in this paper is, of course, mine.

REFERENCES

Basch, Michael Franz (1989) The teacher, the transference and development. In *Learning and Education: Psychoanalytic Perspectives.* Madison: International Universities Press. 1989. eds. Field, Kay, Cohler, Bertram and Wool, Glorye.

Hirschhorn, Larry (1988). *The Workplace Within: Psychodynamics of Organizational Life.* Cambridge: MIT Press.

Klein, Melanie (1936/1964). Love, guild and reparation. In *Love, Hate and Reparation.* New York: Norton.

Welsh, Patrick (1987). *Tales Out of School: A Teacher's Candid Account from the Front Lines of the American High School.* New York: Penguin Books.

Winnicott, D. W. (1965). *The Maturational Processes and the Facilitating Environment.* New York: International Universities Press.